Routledge
Taylor & Francis Group
711 Third Avenue
New York, NY 10017

Routledge
Taylor & Francis Group
27 Church Road
Hove, East Sussex BN3 2FA

© 2012 by Taylor Francis and National Board for Certified Counselors
Routledge is an imprint of Taylor & Francis Group, an Informa business

Printed in the United States of America on acid-free paper
Version Date: 2011916

International Standard Book Number: 978-0-415-88123-4 (Hardback)

Visit the Taylor & Francis Web site at
http://www.taylorandfrancis.com

and the Routledge Web site at
http://www.routledgementalhealth.com

THIRTEENTH EDITION

COUNSELOR PREPARATION

PROGRAMS, FACULTY, TRENDS

Wendi K. Schweiger, Donna A. Henderson, Kristi McCaskill, Thomas W. Clawson, and Daniel R. Collins

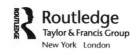

Routledge
Taylor & Francis Group
New York   London

OK copy

Contents

SECTION A   *Purpose and Design*

SECTION B   Related Professional Organizations and Program Structures

SECTION C   Counselor Preparation Programs

Preface

As we submit this *Counselor Preparation* manuscript for publication, we are already discussing ideas for the next book. We are pleased to be continuing the tradition of a process begun by Joe Hollis and Richard Wantz. Many years ago, coauthor Tom Clawson asked Joe Hollis what would happen with the book after Dr. Hollis retired and sold his publishing house, Accelerated Development. Dr. Hollis answered that he would love to see the National Board for Certified Counselors (NBCC) take on a role as copublisher with what is now Routledge of the Taylor & Francis group. NBCC boards continue to support this joint copyright as a service to the profession rather than as a financial venture.

For this edition, we had a lower than usual response rate from programs within the U.S. This is leading us to explore ways with Routledge to improve response, and we hypothesize that the book format will change greatly in the 14th edition.

This is the second edition that has included data from programs outside the U.S. We created a separate survey specifically geared to gathering better data from programs outside the U.S., including space for more open-ended responses and space to indicate counseling training at the undergraduate level, which is considered the appropriate level of training in many countries. Some programs in countries that did not respond for the last edition responded for the first time for this one. We hope that the number of programs responding from other countries will continue to grow. Also included in this edition is a chapter about international counseling students studying in the United States and counseling training in Central and South America. Plans in future editions include inviting authors to submit chapters about counseling in their regions of the world.

This manuscript also includes invited chapters from guest authors covering a variety of topics pertinent to counselor education and the profession as a whole. We started a tradition by inviting guest authors in other parts of the world to write about counseling for the 12th edition, and we thought expanding these invitations to contribute would enrich the 13th edition.

With permission from the Council for Accreditation of Counseling and Related Educational Programs (CACREP) to use their logo, we have continued to indicate the counseling programs that are accredited by CACREP. We have also continued noting the percentages of professors and teaching staff members who are National Certified Counselors (NCCs) to assist students in evaluating faculties that model counselor professionalism. We know that other professionals have dedicated their careers to training counselors. We also know that counseling has become a fully vibrant and separate profession. To that end, we continue to note faculty members who identify themselves as counselors first, and we especially welcome the number of NBCC-certified and state-licensed counselors who work with the next generation of counselors.

We dedicate this edition to the Association for Counselor Education and Supervision for their commitment to quality education and supervision of professional counselors for over 60 years. We appreciate the vision of the many counselors who have helped to develop this important association.

Other plans for the 14th edition will be geared toward ways to expand the response from programs both within the U.S. and outside the U.S. Excerpts from *Counselor Preparation*, 13th Edition, will be posted on the NBCC's Web site at www.nbcc.org.

Wendi K. Schweiger, Ph.D., NCC, LPC
Associate Vice President
NBCC International

Donna A. Henderson, Ph.D., NCC, LPC
Professor
Department of Counseling, Wake Forest University

Kristi McCaskill, M.Ed., NCC, NCSC
Director of Professional Advocacy
National Board for Certified Counselors, Inc. & Affiliates

Thomas W. Clawson, Ed.D., NCC, NCSC, LPC
President and CEO
National Board for Certified Counselors, Inc. & Affiliates

A Tribute to the Association for Counselor Education and Supervision: 60 Years of Dedication to Excellency in Counselor Education and Supervision

It has been almost 60 years since the Association for Counselor Education and Supervision (ACES) assisted in founding the American Counseling Association (ACA) and began dedicating itself to counselor preparation and supervision with the overall effect of enhancing the profession. ACES has continually grown and developed as the division of ACA dedicated to excellence in educating and supervising counselors. ACES serves a vital purpose for professional counseling by focusing on effective preparation and supervision. With an organizational structure that includes elected officers, a general assembly, regional committees, task forces, and a variety of interest networks, ACES works to promote its central mission while also integrating related issues important to counselor education.

ACES' history includes a multitude of counselors who have been involved in developing this organization. We recognize those professionals who have dedicated parts of their careers to volunteering countless hours in supporting this important association and in turn adding leadership and excellence to our profession.

Throughout its history, ACES has demonstrated an ongoing commitment and ability to adapt to and anticipate necessary changes in the education of counselors as the world has changed. ACES leadership has recognized that practice must change to keep pace with an evolving society. The authors of this 13th edition of *Counselor Preparation* dedicate this publication to ACES and to the thousands of professors and supervisors involved in the evolution of this dynamic membership organization.

Introduction: ACES—Past to Present

Thomas Scofield
ACES President (2009–2010)

The Association for Counselor Education and Supervision (ACES) has a long transformational history, spanning almost seven decades. Although certainly changing with the times, ACES has established itself through a strong identity and ever-growing vitality.

HISTORY

ACES began in the early 1940s with a specific focus on guidance and career counseling. It has evolved to encompass rapidly changing technologies, evolving standards, and curricular demands. ACES has demonstrated resilience and owes its identity to responsive leadership, the demands of an ever-increasing multicultural society and complex needs of the diverse publics it serves.

Given the depth of involvement by many, an informative presentation on the history of ACES would be a formidable task as the change and growth of ACES is as varied as it is diverse and is too far-reaching for the limits of this introduction. For a more comprehensive and definitive history, see Elmore (1985) and Sheeley (1977, 1990). The aim of this introduction, therefore, will be to mention briefly some of the major turning points in the history and development of ACES as an association. Secondly, it will provide a description about the association's intended purpose. Additionally, it will detail how the existing structure and governance of the organization relates to the attainment of its goals and objectives. Finally, the introduction concludes with discussion of how the past and present inform the future of our association.

In the earliest of years the association was named the National Association for Guidance and Supervision (NAGS). Name changes of the association seemed to follow approximately every ten years as membership foci, function and involvement shifted. The association's name underwent modification again in the early 1950s becoming the National Association of Guidance Supervisors and Counselor Trainers (NAGSCT) and then again in the early 1960s when the Association for Counselor Education and Supervision (ACES) constitution was approved (Elmore, 1985). The multiple name changes, however, do little to capture the turbulent nature and staunch leadership required of the times. Without a doubt the seedbed for historical development, according to Elmore, rested with the issues related to program accreditation in the late 1970s; membership attitudes, accountability, and reorganization in the 1980s; and the need for greater solidarity. These became the pivotal aspects surrounding change and the foundational tasks undertaken as members established continuity of strength and vitality for the organization.

PURPOSE

The Mission Statement of ACES is

> As a division of the American Counseling Association (ACA) the mission of the Association for Counselor Education and Supervision (ACES) is to enhance the practice of professional counseling through the promotion of effective counselor education and supervision. ACES advances the generation and dissemination of knowledge that is responsive and respectful of our increasingly diverse world. (ACES, n.d.)

In addition, according to the Bylaws of ACES:

> The purpose of the Association, in accordance with the purpose of ACA, shall be to advance counselor education and supervision in order to improve guidance, counseling and student personnel services in all settings of society. The Association is organized and operated exclusively for charitable and educational purposes within the meaning of section 501(c)(3) of the Internal Revenue Code of 1954 (Article I: Section 3, p. 2, ACES, 2006).

Each of the above statements offers much in the way of appreciating the broader nature of what ACES intends, desires, and thus aspires to accomplish. In 2003, during the ACES Business Meeting, the Executive Council unanimously adopted a vision statement that encompasses and forwards the elements of these positions. This assertion established that our association would be recognized as the "vanguard of change" within the counseling profession. ACES would take a leadership role and commit itself to the advancement of "pedagogy related to the education and training of counselors, supervisors, and counselor educators." In addition, ACES would be guided by its commitment to "(a) affirm and deliver education and supervision related to counseling in a culturally diverse society; (b) promote a unified professional identity for counselors, supervisors, and counselor educators; and (c) provide and disseminate premier research and scholarship" (ACES, 2003). These guiding principles can be found in the 2007 ACES Strategic Plan (ACES, 2007) in which they are tied to specific, measurable, attainable outcomes, thus ensuring cohesiveness and continuity of the association's efforts to reach its goals.

ORGANIZATIONAL STRUCTURE AND GOVERNANCE

The organizational structure of ACES has both expanded and contracted to meet the needs of its members, fiduciary responsibilities and general organizational enterprise. As a division of ACA:

> ACES maintains a separate yet integrated governance structure consisting of elected officers, a General Assembly, regional committees, bylaws, operating procedures, and representatives to the ACA Governing Council (ACES, 2009).

The overview of the ACES Policy and Procedures Handbook and part of the revised ACES Bylaws (April 2006) provide the framework for governing the internal affairs of the association. The actual governance by and through the Executive Council and Executive Committee and ACES State Divisions and Regions has changed very little over the years. Officers serve their respective term according to the established state, regional or national organization bylaws. The standing committees provide ongoing support and direction to the association. These committees include Awards, Budget and Finance, State Division and Strategic Planning, Bylaws and Resolutions, Membership, Nominations and Elections, Product Development and Research Grants.

Currently the task force of Social Justice and Human Rights, ACES/NCDA Joint Commissions for Career Development, and Ethics/Professional Issues make up the special groups designed to address issues germane to the goals and objectives of ACES. In addition, the elected, three-year term of the Governing Council Representative provides a pivotal role that carries the voice (e.g., perspectives, issues and concerns) of the membership to and from ACA.

Finally, the interest networks concerned with Advocacy, College Student Affairs, International Counseling, Clinical Mental Health, Multicultural Interests, New Faculty, Rural Counselors, School Counselors, Technology, Women's Interest and Mentoring, Supervision, Doctoral Programs, Clinic Directors, and Counselor Education Qualitative Research attract members who have a concentrated interest and passion in one or more of these specific areas. The chairs of such committees serve for one year (typically providing mentorship) and may be reappointed if the work of the network is seen as serving the greater good of the association. Thus the organizational flow of all elected roles, committees, groups, and networks provides a governing structure that represents the professional interests of the association at state, regional, national and international levels.

THE FUTURE OF ACES

The future of ACES can be captured in the following phrase: "one journey; multiple paths." The direction of ACES rests with no one person, group, or executive council member past or present. Rather it is shaped by the demands and obligations that the association accepts as its responsibility and charge. To remain viable and relevant, ACES, in its role as the "vanguard of change," must be intentional while embracing greater transparency and inclusiveness. In his *ACES Challenges: Past President's Comments,* Vernon Sheeley (1990b) offered the following:

> Almost everything else in the counseling field depends upon the graduates of those [counselor education] preparation programs—the alumni who are the heart of the profession. Therefore, ACES members need to reexamine, refocus, and rebuild their curricula and continually reach toward higher standards of performance. Members dare not build a curriculum and leave it standing long. It has to be recreated for each new generation of students, for each student, and for those already practicing their trades within ever-shifting and evolving waves of societal development. (p. 239)

As we approach the year 2012, our association's future is most assuredly tied to the fertile and vibrant past. Elmore (1985) advanced the descriptions of Sheeley's six general identified concerns of 20 living presidents whose terms spanned from 1940 to 1977. The areas of concern were

- high priority to professional leadership, conceptualization, and research;
- heeding social forces and occupational trends in counselor education program development;
- recruitment and selection of graduate students in counseling and the quality of counselor preparation programs;
- broader membership and scope of responsibility for the preparation and supervision of counselors in the community;
- fostering motivation for the personal re-education, professional renewal and association development; and
- counselor education standards, accreditation of counselor education programs and credentialing (certification and licensure).

It is astounding how apropos these concerns relate to the vision, mission, existing strategic plan and current focus of ACES.

With these historical underpinnings in mind, ACES should take every advantage and opportunity to invite, mentor and involve emerging leaders who accept the mantle of "stewardship" for shaping the future direction of the association. Now, as in the past, ACES will need to examine evolving trends related to licensure, supervision, counselor education and training with an ever-increasing focus on the quality of counselor preparation and ongoing research that informs its pedagogy and practice. It is essential that ACES demonstrate leadership with regard to innovative methods of training and instruction that pay closer attention to social and professional advocacy, social justice, and multicultural and diversity competencies as well as spirituality and wellness initiatives. Such consideration will reshape programs and ask that we strike a creative balance between technology, the relevance of what is learned, the rigor of our standards and the very human relational elements of our practice and profession.

REFERENCES

Association for Counselor Education and Supervision (2003). *ACES Vision Statement*. Retrieved November 19, 2010, from http://www.acesonline.net/about-aces/documents-minutes/

Association for Counselor Education and Supervision (2006). *ACES Bylaws*. Retrieved November 19, 2010, from http://www.acesonline.net/about-aces/documents-minutes/

Association for Counselor Education and Supervision (2007). *ACES Strategic Plan*. Retrieved November 19, 2010, from http://www.acesonline.net/about-aces/documents-minutes.

Association for Counselor Education and Supervision (2009). *ACES Policy and Procedures Handbook*. Retrieved November 19, 2010, from http://www.acesonline.net/about-aces/documents-minutes/

Association for Counselor Education and Supervision (n.d.). *ACES Mission Statement*. Retrieved November 19, 2010, from http://www.acesonline.net/about-aces/documents-minutes/

Elmore, T. M. (1985). The era of ACES: Tradition, transformation, and the possible dream. *Journal of Counseling and Development, 63*, 411-415.

Sheeley, V. L. (1977). *Presidential review: ACES leaders create ties, 1940–77*. Washington, D.C.: Association for Counselor Education and Supervision.

Sheeley, V. L. (1990a). Five decades of ACES: Service to members. *Counselor Education and Supervision, 29*, 228-238.

Sheeley, V. L. (1990b). ACES challenges: Past president's comments. *Counselor Education and Supervision, 29*, 239-250.

Sheeley, V. L. (1990c). ACES beyond fifty: Creating a future. *Counselor Education and Supervision, 29*, 251-257.

Acknowledgments

The authors begin by thanking the board of directors of the National Board for Certified Counselors, Inc. & Affiliates (NBCC) for their continued support of this publication as a service to the counseling profession. Thank you to all of the counselors from the United States and abroad who took time from teaching, research and working with clients to fill out the surveys that provide the base for the data in this publication. The 12th edition marked the first time that the authors surveyed programs outside of the United States, and we have continued this tradition in this 13th edition.

We are very grateful to the many members of NBCC staff who assisted in this project. Their expertise is vital to the publication of *Counselor Preparation*. Dan Collins used his extensive expertise to create two surveys, one for domestic programs and one for programs outside the U.S. With his experience as both a counselor and counselor educator combined with his knowledge of computer programming, we are fortunate that he is involved in this edition.

We appreciate Adriana Petrini for her expertise and for assisting with data analysis; Adriana, Bellah Kiteki, Mary Frazier and Joe Wilkerson for their assistance in editing; and Gayle McCorkle and Vivian Mock for their overall assistance. Thank you to Cristina Lima for her work toward creating and testing the survey. We are grateful to Jim Buice for his extensive editing of this edition as it developed.

We would also like to express our sincere gratitude to our guest authors Carol Bobby and Robert Urofsky, Sandra Lopez-Baez, Kok-Mun Ng and Jared Lau, Tom Scofield, and Tom Sweeney. We believe that their contributions helped to more fully address multiple aspects of counselor education in this country and outside it.

To all who contributed their time, energy and ideas, we are deeply grateful.

Purpose and Design

Chapter 1

The Profession

Early editions of this book aimed to provide a reference of counselor education programs, faculty members, and emerging trends, and over the years, *Counselor Preparation* has expanded to help students research and learn about the variety of programs available. In order to best understand the counseling program as it currently exists, this book opens with a discussion of the beginnings of the counseling profession.

MILESTONES IN THE HISTORY OF COUNSELING

Around the turn of the 20th century, the counseling profession emerged from a growing awareness of people's need for guidance in personal, vocational and academic matters. While the settings of these services were diverse, the goal of helping people face challenges constructively was an early, fundamental purpose. One of the earliest proponents of this movement was Jesse B. Davis, a Detroit principal who established the first guidance program in public schools. Later, in 1908, Clifford Beers advocated for better facilities and treatment for the mentally ill in his book, *A Mind That Found Itself.* That same year, Frank Parsons founded the Boston Vocational Bureau, a place designed to help young people find jobs. World Wars I and II extended the need for counselors through the emphasis on psychological testing for military recruitment. In these early years, several people influenced the developing profession, including Lightner Witmer, Morris S. Viteles, Alfred Binet, G. Stanley Hall and even Sigmund Freud.

Before counseling could be considered a profession, specific criteria had to be met. These include

1. Specific body of knowledge with recognized training programs. To be considered a profession, a body of knowledge must be accumulated in the area. One indication of this accomplishment is that by 1964, the U.S.

Department of Health, Education, and Welfare listed 327 institutions of counselor preparation.

2. Professional organization of peers. Early examples of this occurred in 1913 and 1914 with the formation of the National Vocational Guidance Association and the National Association of Deans of Women (later named the National Association of Women Deans and Counselors). Now the counseling profession has more than 30 professional associations and specialties in the field.

3. Accreditation of training programs. This criterion was met with the establishment of the Council for Accreditation of Counseling and Related Educational Programs (CACREP) in 1981. CACREP helps ensure the quality of counselor education training programs by recognizing programs meeting defined standards.

4. Supervised clinical training. In addition to extensive classroom instruction, clinical training under the supervision of qualified professional practitioners is required in the education of counselors. The amount of clinical experience is measured in clock hours, with the required number steadily increasing as the profession has advanced.

5. Certification of practitioners. Certification refers to the process of earning a credential from a professional organization. The certification affirms that a board of professionals in an area of specialization has reviewed a person's qualifications and found that the individual meets predetermined training and experience requirements. One example of a national certification organization for counselors is the National Board for Certified Counselors (NBCC), which was created in 1982. Today, NBCC provides national counselor certifications and recognizes individual counselors who meet established professional standards.

6. Legal recognition and licensure. State and federal laws and acts have created qualification standards and practice limits for counselors in private practice. A licensure law stipulates who can call themselves counselors and what functions they can perform. This legal recognition enhances the level of professionalism. State licensure laws for counseling exist in all 50 states, the District of Columbia, Guam, and Puerto Rico.

MAJOR STEPS TO BECOMING A PROFESSIONAL COUNSELOR IN THE UNITED STATES

To enter the profession of counseling, a person must

1. Graduate with a baccalaureate degree from a regionally accredited institution of higher education.
2. Be accepted to a graduate degree program in counseling. The selection of the program may depend on several considerations, including

program location, desired specialty area, program accreditation and faculty credentials.

3. Complete a graduate degree program in counseling. The number of academic hours varies by program and institution. The minimum is generally 48 graduate-level academic semester hours, which may include hours for practicum and internship.

4. Complete a practicum. Designed to assist in the acquisition of basic skills, the practicum experience allows students to extend the knowledge acquired from academic coursework and provides supervised opportunities to apply techniques. The number of clock hours required varies with the program.

5. Complete a supervised clinical internship. Internship experiences continue the development of skills and techniques under supervision and prepare students to assume employment in the field. The number of clock hours required, the type of setting and the amount of supervision varies from program to program.

6. Graduate from the counselor program with a master's degree or higher.

7. Apply for national certification and state licensure. National certification recognizes professionals who have met established standards based on research whereas licensure provides legal authorization to practice in a particular state.

THE COUNSELING PROFESSION

Counselors use professional knowledge and skills to assist people who are experiencing life changes. Counselors may help others with concerns that include stress, loss, career, relationships and other personal issues. Some individuals may be struggling with mental illnesses while others are dealing with common life changes. In all situations, counselors focus on the person's stage of life and abilities to cope with life changes and challenges.

REFERENCE

Beers, C.W. (1943). *A mind that found itself*, 3rd ed. Garden City, NY: Doubleday, Doran & Company.

Chapter 2

Credentialing of Counselors

Before officially enrolling, students often consider counselor education programs which provide rich opportunities to develop skills, expectations and interests. Researching each program and comparing several closely will help students identify and select challenging academic experiences, which will in turn lead to satisfying professional environments. Factors affecting a student's selection of a program vary and may include considerations such as cost, geographic location, size, campus appearance, recommendations from family or friends and the availability of financial aid. However, astute students also gather detailed information about post-graduation credentialing opportunities from each program they are considering. Students may be eligible to obtain professional counseling credentials after graduation although the program's length or requirements are critical determinants.

Credentials raise a counselor's level of professional respect among peers, clients, the community and colleagues. In most cases, obtaining credentials indicates that a counselor has been reviewed by a professional board and has successfully completed predetermined standards. Credential sources include education, membership organizations, state licensure and national certification.

EDUCATION

One of the main types of credentials is an academic degree. While academic degrees include bachelor's programs, the completion of graduate degree in counseling is the basis for practice as a professional counselor in the United States. Graduate coursework in counseling may be at the master's, specialist or doctoral level. Generally speaking, a master's degree requires the completion of a 48- or 60-semester-hour program while specialist programs are designed for people who wish to augment skills in pursuit of advanced certifications or other professional objectives. In the United States, doctoral degrees in counselor education are generally designed for those interested in conducting research or teaching. Many recognize the more advanced degrees (i.e., a Ph.D. compared with an M.A.) as the stronger of the credentials; however, other factors are also significant to an individual's academic credentials. These factors include the reputations of the academic department and college or university and the accreditation of programs from organizations such as the Council for Accreditation of Counseling & Related Educational Programs (CACREP). Please see Chapter 6 for more details regarding CACREP.

Another important consideration in regards to academic credentials is the major area of study or specialization. Typically, the area of specialization should match with the counselor's area of practice. For example, an M.A. in counseling with a specialization in school counseling would be more relevant in a school setting than in a community setting. Counselors can also successfully transition to other professional counseling work environments after completing additional training and supervision work.

MEMBERSHIP IN PROFESSIONAL ORGANIZATIONS

Counselors are encouraged to become active members in one or more relevant professional organizations. This involvement helps counselors stay abreast of important issues and avenues of research and allows them to network with colleagues in the profession as well as within areas of specialization. Professional organizations may also recognize qualified members through membership classification.

STATE LICENSURE

Licensure refers to state laws, which identify counselors who have been authorized to provide the services described in the licensure law. Because each is passed separately, the laws differ across states. These differences may include the examination used, scope of practice, title and other requirements. More information about state licensure is found in Chapter 4.

NATIONAL CERTIFICATION

In general, practitioners who hold higher credentials are better respected among their peers, clients, and others with whom they work. National certification also provides an excellent source of professional recognition to the general public. Obtaining certification from a nationally recognized certification board is a significant way for professionals to ensure that they remain well qualified and current in their skills and practices. It is also perhaps the most important way to communicate to potential and current clients and other community members that the counselor is well trained and has completed standards based on research in the profession. The National Board for Certified Counselors (NBCC) is the largest national certification organization in counseling. More information about NBCC is found in Chapter 7.

Chapter 3

Research Design and Data Sources

Over the years, the research published in *Counselor Preparation* has evolved, and previous editions formed the outline for the research design and data sources for this edition. A survey that was originally paper-and-pencil has transformed into an online format incorporating technological advancements now available. Following in this chapter are page examples of the survey as it was presented in the online format for this edition.

DATA COLLECTION PROCEDURE

In January 2010, U.S. institutions having counseling master's, specialist and doctoral degrees in the counseling field were invited to complete the online version of the Data Collection Form (see Figure 3.1). As in the past, many additions, deletions and formatting changes were made. The previous edition contained the first attempt at soliciting data collection from international programs and served to better inform the survey creation for all counselor education and training venues. This edition expands the study of counseling training programs outside the United States, which in February 2010 were invited to complete a separate online survey specifically designed for international programs. (See Figure 3.2.)

A list of institutions in the United States with counselor education programs was compiled from an extensive list that NBCC maintains for business purposes, including testing and certification of counselors. NBCC regularly updates this resource. In addition, counseling venues from outside the United States were compiled from a list that is maintained by NBCC International, a division of NBCC.

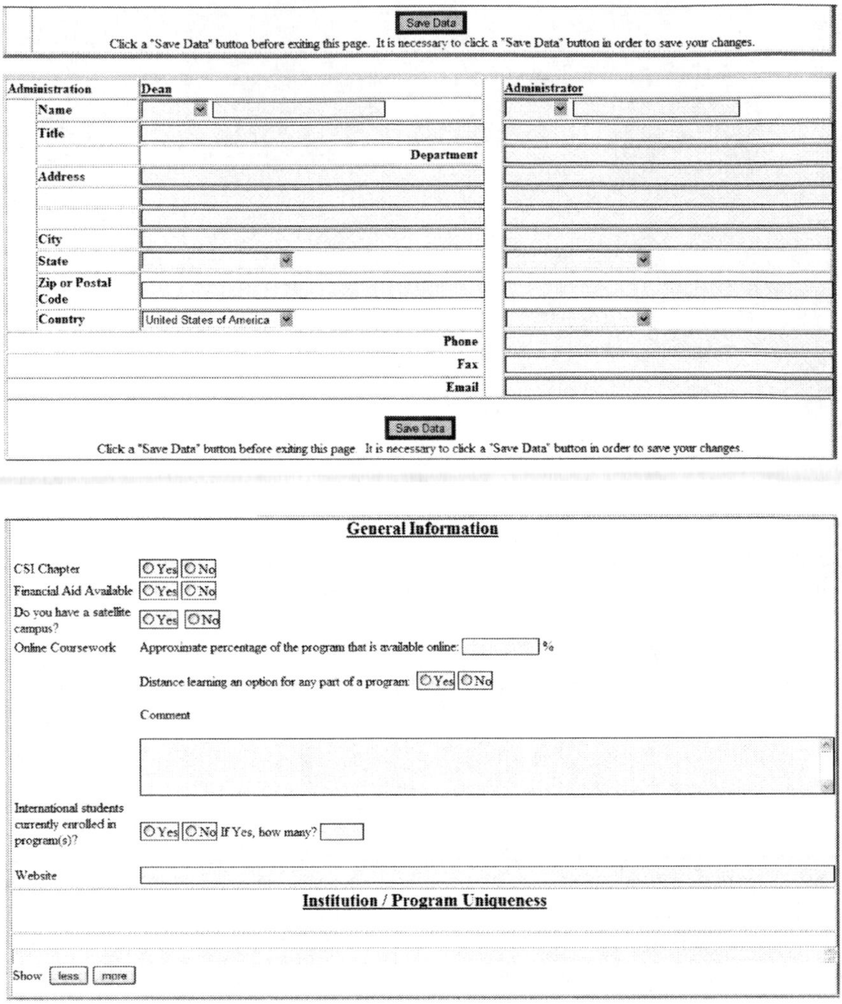

FIGURE 3.1 Excerpts from the Data Collection Form—U.S. Programs.

:k the 'Save Data' button before leaving this page or entered data will be lost.

gram Information

Name	
Contact Person	_Select "Other" to add a person not listed._
Degree	
Admitted Yearly	Number only
Graduated Yearly	Number only
Female Enrollment	Number only
Male Enrollment	Number only
Average Age of Enrolled Student	Number only

Save Data

Click a 'Save Data' button before exiting this page. It is necessary to click a 'Save Data' button in order to save your changes.

Add Faculty

Click a "Save Data" button before exiting this page. It is necessary to click a "Save Data" button in order to save your changes.

Name

    First

    Middle or MI

    Last

    Suffix

Education

    Highest Degree   Select

Academic Position

    Rank   Select

    Instructional Time   Select

Credential

    State Licensed Counselor   ○ Yes ○ No

    NCC   ○ Yes ○ No

FIGURE 3.1 (continued).

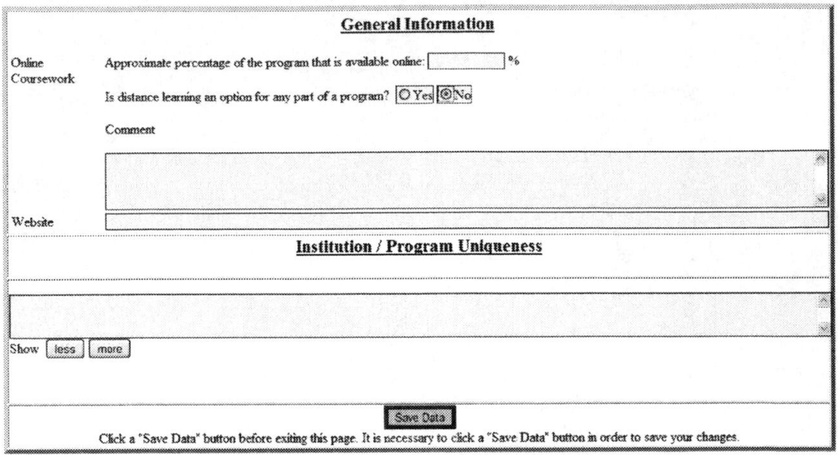

FIGURE 3.2 Excerpts from the Data Collection Form—Programs Outside the U.S.

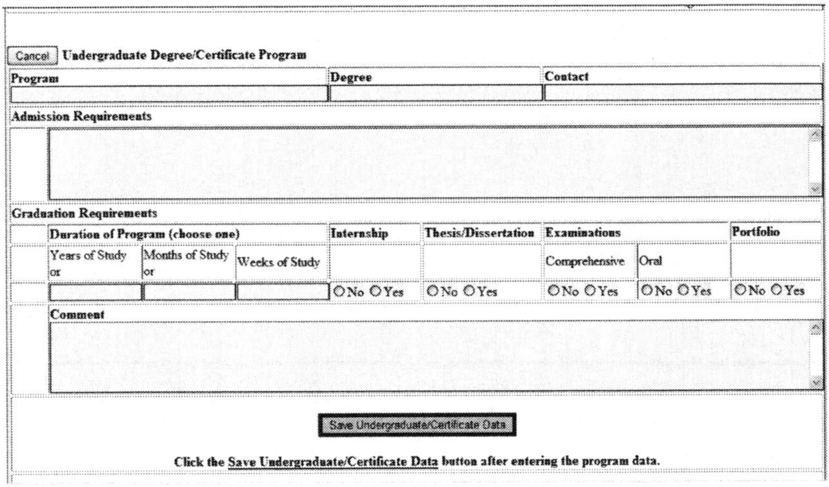

| Cancel | Undergraduate Degree/Certificate Program |

Program	Degree	Contact

Admission Requirements

Graduation Requirements

Duration of Program (choose one)			Internship	Thesis/Dissertation	Examinations		Portfolio
Years of Study or	Months of Study or	Weeks of Study			Comprehensive	Oral	
			○ No ○ Yes	○ No ○ Yes	○ No ○ Yes	○ No ○ Yes	○ No ○ Yes

Comment

Save Undergraduate/Certificate Data

Click the Save Undergraduate/Certificate Data button after entering the program data.

FIGURE 3.2 (continued).

When an institution of higher education houses counseling programs in more than one department, each program is treated distinctly. Every effort has been made to include all counselor preparation units. The authors invite any new or unlisted programs to participate in future surveys. If programs have not previously participated and would like to be included in future research, please contact the National Board for Certified Counselors.

Chapter 4

State Licensure

As of April 2011, state licensure laws exist in all 50 states, the District of Columbia, Guam and Puerto Rico. Counselors should consider the state or states where they might want to practice and become familiar with the specific requirements of that entity. Not only do rules vary between states, they can also vary within any state, depending on the practice setting and specialization. For example, licensure requirements often differ for mental health counselors, school counselors, rehabilitation counselors and student affairs practice professionals. Differences can include the requirements for number of academic semester hours, and the type and amount of clinical experience and supervised clinical practice hours. All states currently use NBCC examinations as a part of licensure requirements.

STATE BOARDS

State boards are the best resources for basic information and current regulations. The contact information for each state board as well as Washington, D.C., Guam, and Puerto Rico as of 2011 is listed below.

Alabama *Law passed 1979.* Dr. Walter H. Cox, Executive Officer, Alabama Board of Examiners in Counseling, 950 22nd St. N, Suite 765, Birmingham, AL 35203-5305; (205) 458-8716; email: walter.cox@abec. alabama.gov; Web site: http://www.abec.state.al.us

Alaska *Law passed 1998.* Ms. Eleanor Vinson, Licensing Examiner, Board of Professional Counselors, Division of Corporations, Business, and Professional Licensing, P.O. Box 110806, Juneau, AK 99811-0806; (907) 465-2551; email: eleanor_vinson@alaska.state.ak.us; Web site: http://www.dced.state.ak.us/occ/ppco.htm

Arizona *Law passed 1988.* Ms. Debra Rinaudo, Executive Director, Arizona Board of Behavioral Health Examiners, 3443 N. Central Ave., Suite 1700, Phoenix, AZ 85012-2201; (602) 542-1864; email: information@azbbhe.us; Web site: http://www.azbbhe.us

Arkansas *Law passed 1979.* Dr. Ann K. Thomas, Executive Director, Arkansas Board of Examiners in Counseling, P.O. Box 70, Magnolia, AR 71754-0070; (870) 901-7055; email: arboec@sbcglobal.net; Web site: http://www.state.ar.us/abec

California *Law passed 2009.* Board of Behavioral Sciences, 1625 N. Market Blvd., Suite S-200, Sacramento, CA 95834; (916) 574-7830; email: bbswebmaster@bbs.ca.gov; Web site: http://www.bbs.ca.gov

Colorado *Law passed 1988.* Ms. Joan Seggerman, Licensing Supervisor, CO State Board of Licensed Professional Counselor Examiners, 1560 Broadway, Suite 1350, Denver, CO 80202-5146; (303) 894-7800; email: Joan.Seggerman@dora.state.co.us; Web site: http://www.dora.state.co.us/registrations

Connecticut *Law passed 1997.* Department of Public Health - State of Connecticut, 410 Capitol Ave. MS #12APP, P.O. Box 340308, Hartford, CT 06134-0308; (860) 509-7603; Web site: http://www.ct-clic.com

Delaware *Law passed 1987.* Ms. Sharianne Eley, Administrative Specialist II, Board of Professional Counselors of Mental Health, 861 Silver Lake Blvd., Canon Building, Suite 203, Dover, DE 19904; (302) 744-4500; email: customerservice.dpr@state.de.us; Web site: http://www.dpr.delaware.gov/boards/profcounselors

District of Columbia *Law passed 1992.* Ms. Gabrielle Schultz, Health Licensing Specialist, D.C. Department of Health, Health Professional Licensing Administration, Board of Professional Counseling, 899 North Capitol St., NE 2nd Floor, Washington, D.C. 20002; (202) 724-8739; email: gabrielle.schultz@dc.gov; Web site: www.hpla.doh.dc.gov/hplasite/default.asp

Florida *Law passed 1981; revised in 1987.* Ms. Cindy Phelps-Dilmore, Regulatory Specialist, Board of Clinical Social Work, Marriage and Family Therapy, and Mental Health Counseling, 4052 Bald Cypress Way, Bin #C08, Tallahassee, FL 32399-3258; (850) 245-4447; email: Cindy_Phelps@doh.state.fl.us; Web site: http://www.doh.state.fl.us/mqa/491

Georgia *Law passed 1984.* Mr. Brig Zimmerman, Executive Director, Georgia Professional Licensing Board Examination Development and Testing Unit, 237 Coliseum Dr., Macon, GA 31217-2440; (478) 207-1484; Web site: http://www.sos.state.ga.us/plb/counselors

Guam *Law passed 1989.* Department of Public Health & Social Services, The Guam Board of Allied Health Examiners, P.O. Box 2816, Agana, GU 96910; (671) 734-7295

Hawaii *Law passed 2005.* DCC-PVL, Attn: MHC, P.O. Box 3469, Honolulu, HI 96801-3469; (808) 586-3000; email: counselor@dcca.hawaii.gov; Web site: http://www.hawaii.gov/dcca/areas/pvl/programs/mental

Idaho *Law passed 1982.* Ms. Deborah Sexton, Technical Records Specialist, Idaho Licensing Board of Professional Counselors and Marriage and Family Therapists, 700 W State St., Boise, ID 83702; (208) 334-3233; email: Deborah.sexton@ibol.idaho.gov; Web site: https://ibol.idaho.gov/IBOL/BoardPage.aspx?Bureau=COU

Illinois *Law passed 1992.* Department of Financial & Professional Regulation, Division of Professional Regulation, 320 W. Washington St., 3rd Floor, Springfield, IL 62786-0002; (217) 782-0458; Web site: http://www.idfpr.com

Indiana *Law passed 1997.* Ms. Valerie Jones, Board Director, Behavioral Health and Human Services Licensing Board, Indiana Professional Licensing Agency, 402 W. Washington St., Room W072, Indianapolis, IN 46204-2298; (317) 234-2064; email: pla5@pla.in.gov; Web site: http://www.in.gov/pla/2885.htm

Iowa *Law passed 1991.* Ms. Judith Manning, Board Executive, Iowa Board of Behavioral Science, Lucas State Office Building, 312 E. 12th Street, Des Moines, IA 50319-9010; (515) 281-4422; Web site: http://www.idph.state.ia.us/licensure/board_home.asp?board=be

Kansas *Law passed 1987.* Ms. Maryann Peerenboom, Credentialing Assistant/Applications, Behavioral Sciences Regulatory Board, 712 S. Kansas Ave., Topeka, KS 66603-3817; (785) 296-3240; email: maryann.peerenboom@bsrb.state.ks.us; Web site: http://www.ksbsrb.org

Kentucky *Law passed 1996; revised 2000.* Ms. Carolyn Benedict, Board Administrator, Kentucky Board of Licensed Professional Counselors, P.O. Box 1360, Frankfort, KY 40602-1360; (502) 564-3296; email: carolyn.kyler@ky.gov; Web site: http://lpc.ky.gov

Louisiana *Law passed 1987.* Ms. Eddye Boeneke, Director, Licensed Professional Counselors Board of Examiners, 8631 Summa Ave., Baton Rouge, LA 70809-3678; (225) 765-2515; email: lpcboard@eatel.net; Web site: http://www.lpcboard.org

Maine *Law passed 1989.* Ms. Colleen Eugley, Board Clerk, Maine Board of Counseling Professionals, Licensure State House Station # 35, Augusta, ME 04333-0001; (207) 624-8603, (207) 624-8674; email: colleen.a.eugley@maine.gov; counsel.board@maine.gov; Web site: http://www.state.me.us/pfr/professionallicensing/professions/counselors/index.htm

Maryland *Law passed 1985.* Tracy DeShields, Executive Director, Maryland Board of Professional Counselors and Therapists, Metro Executive Center 3rd Floor, 4201 Patterson Ave., Baltimore, MD 21215-2299; (410) 764-4732; Web site: http://www.dhmh.state.md.us/bopc

Massachusetts *Law passed 1987.* Ms. Patricia Breslin, Associate Executive Director, Board of Registration of Allied Mental Health & Human Services Professions, 239 Causeway St., Ste 500, Boston, MA 02114-2140; (617) 727-3080; email: leija.t.meadows@state.ma.us; Web site: http://www.mass.gov/dpl/boards/mh

Michigan *Law passed 1988.* Ms. Lucinda Clark, Manager, Licensing Operations, Michigan Board of Counseling, The Bureau of Health Professions, P.O. Box 30670, 611 W. Ottawa St., Lansing, MI 48909; (517) 335-0918; Web site: http://www.michigan.gov/mdch/0,1607,7-132-27417_27529_27536---,00.html

Minnesota *Law passed 2003.* Ms. Kari Rechtzigel, Executive Director, Minnesota Board of Behavioral Health and Therapy, 2829 University Ave. SE, Suite 210, Minneapolis, MN 55414-3293; (612) 617-2178; email: bbht.board@state.mn.us; Web site: http://www.bbht.state.mn.us

Mississippi *Law passed 1985.* Ms. Ann A. Cox, Executive Director, Mississippi State Board of Examiners for Licensed Professional Counselors, 129 E. Jefferson St., P.O. Box 1497, Yazoo City, MS 39194; (662) 716-3932; Web site: http://www.lpc.state.ms.us

Missouri *Law passed 1985.* Ms. Loree Kessler, Executive Director, Division of Professional Registration Committee for Professional Counselors, 3605 Missouri Blvd., P.O. Box 1335, Jefferson City, MO 65102; (573) 751-0018; email: procounselor@pr.mo.gov; Web site: http://pr.mo.gov/counselors.asp

Montana *Law passed 1985.* Mr. Brian Bowers, Application Specialist, MT Board of Social Work Examiners and Professional Counselors, Department of Commerce Professional and Occupational Licensing Division, 301 S. Park, 4th Floor, P.O. Box 200513, Helena, MT 59620-0513; (406) 841-2392; Web site: http://bsd.dli.mt.gov/license/bsd_boards/swp_board/board.page.asp

Nebraska *Law passed 1986.* Department of Health and Human Services, Division of Public Health, P.O. Box 94986, Lincoln, NE 68509-4986; (402) 471-2117; Web site: http://www.hhs.state.ne.us/crl/mhcs/mental/mentalhealth.htm

Nevada *Law passed 2006.* Mr. Raymond E. Smith, Sr., Executive Director, Board of Examiners for Marriage and Family Therapists and Clinical Professional Counselors, P.O. Box 370130, Las Vegas, NV 89137; (702) 486-7388; Web site: http://marriage.state.nv.us/index.htm

New Hampshire *Certification law passed 1992; licensure law passed 1998.* Ms. Peggy Lynch, New Hampshire Board of Mental Health Practice, 117 Pleasant Street, Concord, NH 03301-3852; (603) 271-6762; email: mlynch@dhhs.state.nh.us; Web site: http://www.state.nh.us/mhpb

New Jersey *Law passed 1993.* Ms. Elaine DeMars, Executive Director, New Jersey Division of Consumer Affairs, State Board of Marriage & Family Therapy Examiners, Professional Counselor Examiners

Committee, P.O. Box 45007, Newark, NJ 07101; (973) 504-6415; Web site: http://www.njconsumeraffairs.gov/mft/

New Mexico *Law passed 1993.* Ms. Eva Baca, Administrator, New Mexico Therapy Practice Board, Regulation & Licensing Department, 2550 Cerrillos Rd., P.O. Box 25101, Santa Fe, NM 87504-5101; (505) 476-4610; email: counselingboard@state.nm; Web site: http://www.rld.state.nm.us/counseling/

New York *Law passed 2002.* Dr. David Hamilton, Executive Secretary, New York State Education Department, Office of the Professions, 89 Washington Ave., 2nd Floor E, Albany, NY 12234-1000; (518) 474-3817; email: mhpbd@mail.nysed.gov; Web site: http://www.op.nysed.gov/home.htm

North Carolina *Registry law passed 1983; licensure law passed 1993.* Ms. Jennifer Robertson, Administrator, North Carolina Board of Licensed Professional Counselors, P.O. Box 1369, Garner, NC 27529-1369; (919) 661 0820; email: ncblpc@mgmt4u.com; Web site: http://www.ncblpc.org

North Dakota *Law passed 1989.* Ms. Marge Ellefson, Executive Secretary, North Dakota Board of Counselor Examiners, 2112 10th Ave. SE, Mandan, ND 58554; (701) 667-5969; email: ndbce@btinet.net; Web site: http://www2.edutech.nodak.edu/ndbce

Ohio *Law passed 1984.* Ms. Rena Elliot, Counselor Licensing Coordinator, Ohio Counselor, Social Worker, Marriage and Family Therapist Board, 50 W. Broad St., Suite 1075, Columbus, OH 43215-5919; (614) 466-6462; Web site: http://cswmft.ohio.gov

Oklahoma *Law passed 1985.* Ms. Nena West, Director, Professional Counselor Licensing Division, Oklahoma State Department of Health, 1000 N.E. 10th St., Oklahoma City, Oklahoma 73117-1299; (405) 271-6030; email: nenaw@health.ok.gov; Web site: http://www.health.ok.gov/program/lpc

Oregon *Law passed 1989.* Ms. Becky Eklund, Executive Director, Oregon Board of Licensed Professional Counselors & Therapists, 3218 Pringle Road SE #250, Salem, OR 97302-6312; (503) 378-5499; email: lpc.lmft@state.or.us; Web site: http://www.oblpct.state.or.us

Pennsylvania *Law passed 1998.* Ms. Sandra Matter, Board Administrator, State Board of Social Workers, Marriage and Family Therapists, and Professional Counselors, P.O. Box 2649, Harrisburg, PA 17105-2649, (717) 783-1389; email: st-socialwork@state.pa.us; Web site: http://www.dos.state.pa.us/bpoa/cwp/view.asp?a=1104&q=433177

Puerto Rico *Law passed 2001.* Ms. Liza Quinones Castro, Administrative Assistant, Puerto Rico Board of Examiners of Professional Counselors, P.O. Box 10200, San Juan, PR 00908-0200; (787) 782-8989; Web site: http://www.salud.gov.pr

Rhode Island *Law passed 1987.* Ms. Dawn Pitochelli, Administrative Officer, Board of Mental Health Counselors/Marriage and Family Therapists, Rhode Island Department of Health Professions Regulation, 3 Capitol Hill, Providence, RI 02908-5097; (401) 222-2828; email: dawn.pitochelli@health.ri.gov; Web site: http://www.health.state.ri.us/hsr/professions/mf_counsel.php

South Carolina *Law passed 1985*; *revised law enacted 1998.* Ms. Kate Cox, South Carolina Department of Labor Licensing Regulations Division, Professional and Occupational Licensing, P.O. Box 11329, Columbia, SC 29211-1329; (803) 896- 4665; email: harrings@llr.sc.gov; Web site: http://www.llr.state.sc.us/pol/counselors

South Dakota *Law passed 1990.* Ms. Joyce Vos, Executive Secretary, South Dakota Board of Examiners for Counselors and Marriage and Family Therapists, P.O. Box 2164, Sioux Falls, SD 57101-2164; (605) 331-2927; email: sdbce.msp@midconetwork.com; Web site: http://www.state.sd.us/dhs/boards/counselor/

Tennessee *Law passed 1984.* Ms. Sherry Owens, Board Administrator, TN State Board of Licensed Professional Counselors, Marital and Family Therapists and Licensed Pastoral Therapists, 227 French Landing, Suite 300, Heritage Place Metro Center, Nashville, TN 37228-1608; (888) 310-4650; email: sherry.owens@tn.gov; Web site: http://health.state.tn.us/Boards/PC_MFT&CPT/

Texas *Law passed 1981.* Ms. Bobbe Alexander, Executive Director, Texas State Board of Examiners of Professional Counselors, P.O. Box 149347, Austin, TX 78714-9347; (512) 834-6658; email: lpc@tdh.state.tx.us; Web site: http://www.dshs.state.tx.us/counselor

Utah *Law passed 1994.* Mr. Richard Oborn, Bureau Manager, Department of Occupational Professional Licensing, 160 E. 300 S, Box 146741, Salt Lake City, UT 84114-6741; (801) 530- 6628; email: doplweb@utah.gov; Web site: http://www.dopl.utah.gov/licensing/professional_counseling.html

Vermont *Law passed 1988.* Ms. Diane LaFaille, Staff Assistant, Secretary of State Office Board of Allied Mental Health Practitioners, National Life Bldg, North FL2, Montpelier, VT 05620-3402; (802) 828-2396; email: dlafaill@sec.state.vt.us; Web site: http://vtprofessionals.org/opr1/allied_mental_health

Virginia *Law passed 1976.* Ms. Catherine Chappell, Virginia Board of Counseling, Department of Health Professionals, 9960 Maryland Drive, Suite 300, Perimeter Center, Henrico, VA 23233- 1484; (804) 367-4610; email: coun@dhp.virginia.gov.; Web site: http://www.dhp.virginia.gov/counseling/

Washington *Law passed 1987.* Karen Stricklett, Credentialing Manager, Washington State Department of Health, License Credentialing, Customer Service Office, Health Systems Quality Assurance, P.O. Box 47877,

Olympia, WA 98504-7877; (360) 236-4700; email: Karen.Stricklett@doh.wa.gov; Web site: http://www.doh.wa.gov

West Virginia *Law passed 1986.* Ms. Roxanne Clay, Program Coordinator, West Virginia Board of Examiners in Counseling, 815 Quarrier Street, Suite 212, Charleston, WV 25301-2650; (800) 520-3852; email: rclay27@msn.com; Web site: http://www.wvbec.org

Wisconsin *Law passed 1992.* Mr. Ryan Zeinert, Licensing Examination Specialist, Wisconsin Department of Regulation Licensing, P.O. Box 8935, Madison, WI 53708-8935; (608) 266-0145; email: web@drl.state.wi.us; Web site: http://drl.wi.gov/prof/coun/def.htm

Wyoming *Law passed 1987.* Ms. Veronica Skoranski, Acting Executive Director, Mental Health Professions Licensure Board, 1800 Carey Avenue, 4th Floor, Cheyenne, WY 82002; (307) 777-3628; email: vskora@state.wy.us; Web site: http://plboards.state.wy.us/mentalhealth/index.asp

Related Professional Organizations and Program Structures

Chapter 5

Academic Preparation
in the United States

In order to be considered a professional counselor an individual must have successfully completed a graduate degree at the master's, specialist or doctoral level. Counselor education programs include specific curricular areas and clinical experiences. Curricular work includes group discussions, examinations, culminating project, thesis or dissertation, and other professional activities such as teaching, assisting in a classroom, or working on scholarly projects with the faculty and/or acting as a mentor. Clinical experiences provide an opportunity to practice counseling techniques and skills under supervision. Often, this supervised practice may occur in a clinic or laboratory at a college or university, although students may also be placed in community, school or other settings.

PROGRAM ADMINISTRATION

Counselor education programs generally exist within an academic unit that is located in an educational institution, college or university. The academic unit may offer other programs such as psychology, teacher education or human services.

The accreditation(s) granted to the counselor education program or the institution indicates that standards set by the respective accreditation organization have been met. Students who attend accredited programs are likely to receive a more comprehensive perspective and broader educational opportunities. Earning a degree from an accredited program may also provide students with more career options.

Accredited programs often receive higher recognition and enjoy greater prestige and funding, which lead to strengthened educational experiences for students. More extensive resources, better equipment and highly qualified instructors are all possible benefits of attending an accredited program.

COUNSELOR EDUCATION PROGRAM ACCREDITATION

Accreditation of preparation programs in the United States is usually a voluntary process, and the accreditation organizations are independent from federal and state governments. A professional association often establishes the related accreditation. Each accreditation organization establishes criteria to be met by the program. If a department offers more than one program, each must be evaluated separately. Therefore, an institution that offers more than one counselor education program may have some areas that are accredited while others are not. Accreditation is generally awarded for an established time period and must be re-evaluated and renewed on a regular basis.

Obtaining accreditation requires several steps. The department's faculty and staff must first conduct a self-evaluation following accreditation board guidelines. If they believe the department meets the accreditation criteria, they ask the board to proceed with its own evaluation. Often, the board sends a team of professionals to the campus to perform an on-site inspection. The board then reviews the site team's report, makes revisions and, if appropriate, confers its approval.

The time from which the department starts the process until the board's approval is granted is often two or more years. Obligations on the part of the program wishing to be accredited include (a) preparation of the self-study report, (b) application fees, (c) visitation fees, (d) membership fees, and (e) a separate evaluation of each program. Advantages of program accreditation include (a) providing assurance that the program meets high professional standards, (b) ensuring periodic review of the program, (c) assuring applicants that the program meets high standards, (d) offering graduates of the program advantages (e.g., quicker access to licensure), and (e) providing a source of pride for faculty, students, and the college or university as they contribute to or become involved in a nationally recognized program.

COUNSELING ACCREDITATION ORGANIZATIONS

The major accreditation organizations in counseling include the Council for Accreditation of Counseling and Related Educational Programs (CACREP), the Council on Rehabilitation Education (CORE) and the American Association of Pastoral Counselors (AAPC). Each is described below.

Council for Accreditation of Counseling and Related Educational Programs

The largest accreditation board in counseling is the Council for Accreditation of Counseling and Related Educational Programs (CACREP). For more detailed information about CACREP and its history, see Chapter 6.

CACREP is recognized as a specialized accrediting agency by the Council for Higher Education Accreditation. Table 5.1 lists the number of programs accredited in the United States as listed on the Web site as of April 2011 (http://www.cacrep.org/directory/directory.cfm).

Contact information for CACREP:

Council for Accreditation of Counseling and Related Educational Programs
1001 North Fairfax Street, Suite 510
Alexandria, VA 22314
Phone: 703.535.5990
Fax: 703.739.6209
E-mail: cacrep@cacrep.org
Web site: http://www.cacrep.org

Each domestic university/college listing in this edition has been checked against the accreditation list issued by CACREP.

TABLE 5.1 Number of CACREP-Accredited U.S. Programs and Their Classifications/Master's and Doctoral Level

Kind of Program	Number of Programs
Community Counseling	167
Mental Health Counseling	60
Clinical Mental Health Counseling	14
School Counseling	214
College Counseling	17
Student Affairs	25
Career Counseling	9
Marital, Couple, and Family Counseling/Therapy	33
Marriage, Couple, and Family Counseling	3
Gerontological Counseling	1
Counselor Education and Supervision	60

Note: The new standards were passed in 2009. Therefore, CACREP listings currently include programs accredited under both the 2001 and 2009 standards.

Council on Rehabilitation Education

The Council on Rehabilitation Education (CORE) accredits graduate rehabilitation counselor education programs. CORE is recognized by the Council on Higher Education Accreditation and is a member of the Association of Specialized and Professional Accreditors. As of April 2011, the CORE Web site (http://www.core-rehab.org/progrec.html) lists 94 CORE-accredited master's-level rehabilitation programs.

Contact information for CORE:

Council on Rehabilitation Education
1699 Woodfield Road, Suite 300
Schaumburg, IL 60173
Phone: 847.944.1345
Fax: 847.944.1346
Email: sdenys@cpcredentialing.com
Web site: www.core-rehab.org

American Association of Pastoral Counselors

The American Association of Pastoral Counselors (AAPC) was founded in 1963. In addition to certifying pastoral counselors, AAPC accredits pastoral counseling centers and training programs. Pastoral counseling programs can be accredited as training programs, service centers, or both. As of April 2011, the AAPC Web site (http://aapc.org/content/aapc-accredited-centers#AL) lists 17 training programs accredited by AAPC.

Contact information for the AAPC:

American Association of Pastoral Counselors
9504A Lee Highway
Fairfax, VA 22031-2303
Phone: 703.385.6967
Fax: 703.352.7725
E-mail: info@aapc.org
Web site: http://www.aapc.org

FACULTY

Counselor education faculty members provide and supervise academic experiences. Therefore, the qualifications, interests and interpersonal styles of the faculty significantly contribute to the quality of the program. The information that follows introduces some ways to compare faculty contributions across different programs and departments. Summary data presented in this and all data chapters are for U.S. programs only. Programs from outside the United States will be discussed in Chapter 13.

Degrees Held

The total number of faculty members reported from the responding programs was 609. Table 5.2 shows that the majority of them hold terminal degrees, Ph.D. or Ed.D. Over the past 20 years, the percentage of counselor educators with the Ed.D. degree has dropped significantly as many universities have begun to award the Ph.D. instead. Section D in this book contains more faculty information. Table 5.2 also provides a summary of the academic rank of the faculty members. The rank held may not reflect many specifics about a department or about an individual faculty member. Rank may be related to the amount of time a faculty member has taught at an institution of higher education. Rank may also indicate the academic or scholarly contributions made by the faculty member, such as professional publications, research or teaching achievements.

Credentials Held by Faculty

Credentials other than rank and degree provide another measure of faculty qualifications and commitment to the counseling profession. Chapter 2 in this edition explains credentialing. Maintaining credentials usually requires continuing education as well as periodic checks by the state licensing board and the certification organization. A summary of credentials reported for faculty members from responses to the Data Collection Form appears in Table 5.3. Of the 609 faculty members listed, 227 were reported as holding the NCC credential, which represents 37% percent of the total.

TABLE 5.2 Faculty Rank and Degree

Academic Rank	Ph.D.	Ed.D.	Other
Professor Emeritus	4	2	1
Full Professor	122	39	16
Associate	139	23	11
Assistant	149	10	6
Adjunct	25	6	32
Instructor	11	2	10
Lecturer	0	0	1

TABLE 5.3 Summary of NCCs
and State Licenses for Faculty

Number Reported	Credential
322	State Licensed in Counseling
227	NCC-National Certified Counselor

Faculty Time Devoted to Counselor Preparation

In addition to teaching, higher education programs require faculty members to devote time to consulting, supervising and publishing as well as serving on committees. These various duties impact faculty availability and may be an important consideration for certain students selecting a counselor educational program. The amount of available time varies among counseling programs. One way to compute this variable is to compare the assigned faculty time with the number of students in the program. The ratio of student per faculty full-time equivalency (Stu/Fac FTE) is an indicator of faculty availability. The data included in Section D, Data on Each Department, could be used to perform this computation.

Another way to analyze faculty time available is by reviewing the time devoted to counselor preparation programs as reported for this study. The Data Collection Form asked respondents to indicate the percentage of time devoted to counselor preparation programs in one of five groupings: less than 21 percent, 22–40 percent, 41–60 percent, 61–80 percent, and 81–100 percent. Of the 495 responses to this question, 54% indicated faculty time devoted to counselor preparation amounted to more than 61%. These percentages are reported in Table 5.4.

TABLE 5.4 Percentage of Faculty Time Devoted
to Counselor Preparation Programs

0–21%	20%
22–40%	15%
41–60%	10%
61–80%	13%
81–100%	41%
Total responses	495
No responses	186

Degrees Offered

As stated earlier, students in counselor preparation programs in the United States may be pursuing a master's degree, an educational specialist's degree or a doctoral degree. Increasingly, master's programs are offering fifth- or sixth-year programs. Chapter 9 contains summary information about master's degree programs, and Chapter 10 contains summary information about specialist programs. Chapter 11 includes information about doctoral-level study in counselor education. At each level, programs determine admission and graduation criteria as well as the minimum number of academic courses and clinical experiences to include in the program.

Clinical Experience During Training

The clinical experience in counselor preparation programs often occurs in two parts, a practicum and an internship. Typically, the practicum occurs earlier in a program than the internship. Both components require direct supervision by a qualified supervisor in group and/or individual settings. The number of clock hours required for practicum and internship varies from program to program. CACREP standards list the practicum as a 100-hour experience and the internship as a 600-hour requirement. The site for clinical experiences depends on the location of the college or university and the community resources. The goal of most programs is to provide an in-depth experience at a site that has working conditions similar to the student's career goals.

In summary, students may experience a wide variation in academic preparation that can incorporate the administration of the counselor preparation program; its accreditation status; faculty education, rank, credentials and the time devoted to the counseling program; the range of degrees offered; and the clinical experiences.

REFERENCES

American Association of Pastoral Counselors. (n.d.). AAPC accredited centers. Retrieved April 15, 2011, from http://aapc.org/content/aapc-accredited-centers#AL

The Council for Accreditation of Counseling and Related Educational Programs. (n.d.). Directory. Retrieved April 15, 2011, from http://www.cacrep.org/directory/directory.cfm

Council on Rehabilitation Education. (n.d.). Programs recognized: Current. Retrieved April 15, 2011, from http://www.core-rehab.org/progrec.html

Chapter 6

CACREP
Thirty-Something and Aging Well

Carol L. Bobby
CACREP President

Robert I. Urofsky
CACREP Director of Accreditation

Thirty years ago, in 1981, the Council for Accreditation of Counseling and Related Educational Programs (CACREP) incorporated as a nonprofit organization. Since that time, the original purposes outlined in the Articles of Incorporation have served as the cornerstone of CACREP's ability to be successful and maintain steady growth in the number of programs seeking its accreditation. Furthermore, CACREP's reputation and credibility have grown because of its leadership's continued commitment to developing and maintaining accreditation standards that are viable, forward thinking, and based on excellence for the preparation of all counselors.

THE PAST

CACREP's genealogy is traced back to the early 1950s with a connection to the National Association of Guidance Supervisors (NAGS). In 1952, NAGS began to include counselor preparation in its activities and changed its name to the National Association of Guidance Supervisors and Counselor Training

(NAGSCT). As the importance of counselor training issues expanded within this organization's mission, a final name change occurred and the Association for Counselor Education and Supervision (ACES) was born.

Discussions within ACES during the late 1950s and early 1960s fostered a growing support among its membership for standardizing counselor preparation. ACES' first efforts toward achieving such standardization resulted in the development of guidelines for school counselor programs in 1963. Meantime, other organizations, the American School Counselor Association (ASCA) and the American College Personnel Association (ACPA), were developing guidelines and standards for use by their constituent program areas. With so much activity occurring, ACES called for the creation of a joint committee charged to create one set of standards that could be used by *all* programs in counseling and student personnel services. Robert Stripling, credited with being the father of counselor education accreditation, chaired this committee. The instrumental work done by this committee resulted in the adoption of the *ACES Standards for the Preparation of Counselors and Other Personnel Services Specialists* in 1973. This seminal document presented the first set of standards describing the core educational requirements for preparing entry-level professional counselors. With the development of professional standards, there was a concomitant need for the development of processes by which adherence to these standards could be determined.

Under the strong leadership of ACES President Robert (Pete) Havens (1978–79), the ACES Committee on Accreditation was charged to pursue national accreditation efforts. Training sessions on the standards and on-site review processes were held and pilot accreditation visits occurred. However, the involvement of multiple related organizations in ACES' early accreditation efforts created numerous complications as the different groups each had their own priorities for the process. As a result, ACES decided that stronger and more concerted efforts could more readily occur through the umbrella structure of the American Personnel and Guidance Association (APGA), now the American Counseling Association (ACA). In 1980, APGA agreed to adopt the ACES Standards and assist in the creation of an entity responsible for administering an accreditation process based on the standards. These decisions gave birth to the Council for the Accreditation of Counseling and Related Educational Programs (CACREP).

The first meeting of the CACREP Board of Directors took place the following September. The original board structure included representatives from the different groups involved in ACES' early efforts in accreditation. Each division of ACA that wanted to participate in CACREP appointed a leader to represent its interests on the Board. Joseph Wittmer served as CACREP's first Executive Director.

At the initial meeting, the CACREP Board made a commitment to seek external approval of its accreditation review process through the Council on Postsecondary Accreditation (COPA), essentially an accreditor of accrediting groups. The board sought COPA recognition because it believed that committing to an external evaluation and recognition process at the national level would demonstrate to program faculty, higher education administrators, and the public that CACREP intended to operate in the best interest of its constituents. CACREP achieved COPA recognition in 1987 and recognition has been continuously maintained through COPA's successor organizations. Currently, this recognition is granted to CACREP by the Council for Higher Education Accreditation.

THE PRESENT

CACREP is now 30 years old and accredits over 590 counseling programs at over 250 institutions. CACREP's success and ongoing growth is attributable to focused leadership efforts to remain true to its mission, which states the following:

> The mission of CACREP is to promote the professional competence of counseling and related practitioners through the development of preparation standards, the encouragement of excellence in program development, and the accreditation of professional preparation programs (*CACREP Accreditation Manual*, 2009).

Furthermore, CACREP is committed to accomplishing this mission with the understanding that counselor preparation must reflect the changing needs of a diverse and complex society.

There are two key organizational functions that support CACREP's work in fulfilling its mission. First is the structure of the CACREP Board, whose members serve as both the governing board members of the organization and the accreditation decision-making body. The second is the standards revision process.

The CACREP Board

The CACREP Board of Directors ranges from 13 to 15 members. At any given time, at least 8 of these members must be counselor educators, 2 must be counseling practitioners, and 2 must be public members from outside of the counseling profession. This composition allows the board to acknowledge that its primary constituents are counselor education programs, but that input is needed from the practitioner and public constituencies to ensure continued relevancy to what occurs outside academia. The remaining positions may be selected by the board based upon current needs. The board's decision-making process is also of paramount importance to "encourage excellence in program development." (*CACREP Accreditation Manual*, 2009). The CACREP accreditation process involves multiple layers of review from the initial review of an applicant program's self-study, to an on-site visit by a team of trained visitors, to a final board review and accreditation decision. At every level of this process, programs receive feedback from CACREP with regard to how well they meet the CACREP Standards. Programs that have not satisfied the accreditation conditions are given the opportunity to withdraw from the review process without prejudice prior to an adverse decision. Programs that have demonstrated substantial adherence to the CACREP standards but have not satisfied all requirements for a full 8-year accreditation are granted a 2-year accreditation to allow time for minor deficiencies to be remedied and as incentive to continue program improvements. This process has been in place since CACREP's creation and demonstrates CACREP's desire for all programs to strive toward meeting the standards, as well as CACREP's intent to provide fair and thorough reviews.

Standards Revision

The second major function that assists CACREP in meeting its mission is standards revision. Occurring every seven years, the CACREP standards revision process provides an opportunity for CACREP and its constituents to closely examine what is happening in the profession and in society that may require revisions to the counselor preparation standards. The standards revision process ensures that the CACREP Standards remain relevant, so that tomorrow's counselors will have the knowledge and skills necessary to work with the diverse and complex needs of individuals and families in our rapidly changing society.

When standards revision occurs, every CACREP standard is carefully reviewed for continued relevancy and validity, and this allows the revision committee to examine what might be needed for the future. The committee that carries out the revision process is external to the CACREP Board, but keeps the board informed of its findings and revisions. The committee's work is based on a transparent process that includes seeking feedback from counseling professionals and the public, consulting relevant professional literature, and conducting research relevant to the revision process. Public drafts are disseminated at points throughout the process for comment by anyone who wishes to participate.

CACREP's most recent standards revision process culminated in the adoption of the July 2009 CACREP Standards. New areas included in the 2009 Standards are (1) stronger requirements for faculty qualifications; (2) a greater focus on counselors' roles in national emergencies, incidents of trauma, and crisis intervention; (3) evidence that student learning outcomes are defined and measured by programs; and (4) revisions to several program areas offered for accreditation. The 2009 Standards provide program area standards for master's degree programs in the following areas: Addiction Counseling; Career Counseling; Clinical Mental Health Counseling; Marriage, Couple and Family Counseling; School Counseling; and Student Affairs and College Counseling. Additionally, the standards include doctoral degree programs in Counselor Education and Supervision.

THE FUTURE

CACREP is as committed to its future as it is proud of its past. As CACREP enters into its fourth decade of quality assurance reviews, it remains committed to advancing the counseling profession.

Technology has already begun to change the way that counselor preparation occurs. Some counseling students are taking classes on-line and others may be receiving supervision on-line through secure chat rooms with other students or via video Skype with a professor. CACREP has to find ways to determine if students are learning the knowledge and skills necessary to work in tomorrow's counseling settings, regardless of the means by which programs are choosing to deliver course content or supervision. The 2009 Standards are representative of a significant shift away from a sole focus on what is taught to an increased emphasis on programs demonstrating how they ensure students are learning.

Since technology and the information super highway have made contact with peoples from all areas of the world more accessible, CACREP also plans to globalize its mission of advancing the counseling profession through its development of a new quality assurance review process for international counselor education programs. This quality assurance initiative is called the International Registry of Counsellor Education Programs (IRCEP; www.ircep.org). IRCEP's steering committee met for the first time in fall 2009 to develop standards that could be used globally for training counselors regardless of country, culture, or educational degree requirements. The intent of the IRCEP is to create linkages of counselors worldwide that can advance understanding of cultural and educational diversity, while fostering research and student or faculty exchanges. Programs that have successfully completed the IRCEP quality review process will be listed on an international registry.

CACREP is also committed to a future where counselor preparation in the United States is highly regarded by all publics for the education and skills that our graduates bring to a variety of work settings. CACREP is committed to informing school administrators, state departments of education, state counselor licensure boards, and federal legislators why counselor education under the CACREP Standards is appropriate, is thorough, and prepares competent graduates for counseling practice. The future holds excitement for CACREP and its constituents as continued growth is expected.

A SNAPSHOT OF CACREP FACTS

1. CACREP has had only two Chief Executive Officers in its history.
2. Since 1981, CACREP has elected ten chairs to lead the board in its decision-making responsibilities. The current CEO has worked under each of these chairs.

3. There have been four major revisions to the CACREP Standards since adoption of the initial standards—1988, 1994, 2001 and 2009.
4. The eight core curricular areas have been in place since CACREP's inception and with each standards revision process have been reaffirmed as relevant and valid.
5. CACREP has trained over 500 volunteer team members and chairs, of which approximately 340 remain on active status.
6. In 2005, CACREP revised its board membership structure from an appointment-based process relying on ACA and its divisions to a function-based structure relying on the needs of the board to have expertise in specific areas.
7. Since 2008, CACREP has received no financial support from ACA, as compared to the almost 100% reliance on ACA financial support in the early 1980s. While some monetary support is currently provided by the NBCC, CACREP continues to move toward complete financial independence.
8. In 2009, CACREP launched IRCEP by creating an international committee that created the first IRCEP Standards and review processes.
9. In June 2011, CACREP celebrated its 30th anniversary.

REFERENCES

Council for Accreditation of Counseling and Related Educational Programs. *CACREP Accreditation Manual: 2009 Standards* (2009). Alexandria, VA: Author.

Chapter 7

The National Board
for Certified Counselors

The National Board for Certified Counselors (NBCC) was incorporated in 1982 to create a registry of professional counselors. In the early 1980s, counseling as a profession was still developing. In fact, only a small number of states had passed licensure laws regulating the practice of counseling. Influential counseling leaders envisioned the need for a separate organization to provide a national registration and counseling certification system. This represented an important step in the professionalization of counseling, the process whereby an occupation is formalized to enhance the integrity of services provided. (Other indicators of professionalization include specialized accreditation, see Chapter 6; state licensure, see Chapter 4; membership organizations, see A Tribute and Introduction to ACES; standards of conduct; and body of knowledge.) As a result, NBCC was founded in 1982 as an independent, not-for-profit organization which identifies individuals who have voluntarily met research-based, profession-specific requirements.

Very soon after its creation, NBCC became involved in advocacy efforts, stimulated in part by the organization's mission to identify counselors who had met professionally appropriate standards. At that time, there were several states working on obtaining legislation which would regulate the practice of counseling. While legislators were considering the need for licensure, they required facts on the number of professionals involved. NBCC was naturally a good source of this information because the organization had specific information about the number and qualifications of professional counselors by state.

Data about the number and practice of counselors are important, but not the only consideration when creating state licensure laws. Although most licensure boards become self-supporting, it can be costly to set up a licensure process—creation of information sources, identification of board members, development of applications, etc. In particular, the development and maintenance of relevant, research-based examinations can be overwhelming to state governments. Because of national certification, this process had already been completed, and according to rigorous industry standards. Therefore, it was logical to use the examinations developed by NBCC. As of 2011, all fifty states, the District of Columbia, and Puerto Rico use NBCC examinations as part of their state licensure processes. The NBCC examinations used for state licensure include the National Counselor Examination for Licensure and Certification (NCE) and the National Clinical Mental Health Counseling Examination (NCMHCE).

NATIONAL CERTIFICATIONS OFFERED BY NBCC

NBCC's primary purpose is the identification of counselors who meet profession-defined standards. This process allows counselors to distinguish themselves from others who possess only the required license to practice. Pursuing and maintaining national certifications demonstrates a professional commitment to providing quality counseling services. Additionally, possessing national certification(s) affords individual counselors a privilege to use professional designations in communications including letterhead, Web sites, and business cards; and these, in turn, award more public credibility.

Examinations are but one piece of national counseling certifications. In order to determine the requirements of national certification, experts closely examined all aspects of the profession and what exemplified quality counseling practices. Ultimately, these experts identified five features.

Master's-Level Education

It is easy to overlook the fact that counseling in the United States did not begin as a master's-level profession; however, counseling's roots extend back to around the beginning of the twentieth century when leaders realized that students would benefit from having specialized assistance in making educational and vocational decisions. Today, counseling is a master's-level or higher profession.

Specific Coursework

Beyond the level of education, professional counselors must complete coursework in specific areas. These include human growth and development, social and cultural foundations, helping relationships, group work, career and lifestyle development, appraisal, research and program evaluation, and professional orientation and ethics.

Internship Experience

While students are in their graduate programs, they are placed in counseling settings to apply the information and techniques they are learning. These settings are generally related to the student's area of interest such as clinical mental health or school. Internship experiences often start with the student observing a variety of counseling tasks; however, over time, the student is assigned more direct duties which are closely monitored by the student's supervisors.

Supervised Experience

Another requirement for national certification through NBCC is the completion of supervised experience. While supervised experience begins during the counselor education program through internship experiences, candidates for national certification must be able to demonstrate that they have continued developing their counseling skills by working under the supervision of another qualified professional.

National Examination

National counselor examinations developed by NBCC are designed to assess an applicant's knowledge of counseling information deemed appropriate for effective counselor functioning. NBCC examinations are created in adherence to the Standards for Educational and Psychological Testing (1999) and the Uniform Guidelines on Employee Selections Procedures (1978).

THE NATIONAL CERTIFIED COUNSELOR (NCC)

The NCC is the flagship national certification for professional counselors. This certification recognizes those counselors who have voluntarily met the rigorous standards defined by the counseling profession. As of 2011, there are more than 47,000 individuals certified.

All counselors who are interested in obtaining certification through NBCC must

1. Hold a minimum of a master's degree in counseling or a degree with a major study in counseling from a regionally accredited university.
2. Complete a minimum of 48 semester or 72 quarter hours of graduate-level coursework, with at least one course in the above referenced coursework areas.

3. Document two academic terms of supervised field experience in a counseling setting.
4. Document two years of post-master's counseling experience with 3,000 hours of counseling work experience and 100 hours of face-to-face supervision.
5. Provide two professional endorsements, one of which must be from a recent supervisor.
6. Pass an accepted NBCC examination (the NCE or the NCMHCE).

SPECIALTY CERTIFICATIONS

Another advantage of seeking national certification is that this system provides opportunities for counselors to indicate areas of specialty practice. NBCC currently offers three specialization certifications: clinical mental health counseling, school counseling, and addictions counseling. NBCC retired specialty certifications in gerontological counseling and career counseling in 1999.

The Certified Clinical Mental Health Counselor (CCMHC) was created through the merger of the National Academy of Clinical Mental Health Counselors and NBCC and recognizes counselors who have voluntarily met national standards in clinical mental health counseling.

The Master Addictions Counselor (MAC) certification was created by the joint efforts of ACA, the International Association of Addiction and Offender Counselors and NBCC. The MAC certification identifies counselors who meet national professional standards in addictions counseling.

National Certified School Counselor (NCSC) certification recognizes counselors who have specialized knowledge and meet the highest standards of training for the practice of counseling in school settings.

REQUIREMENTS TO MAINTAIN NBCC CERTIFICATIONS

Once counselors successfully complete the requirements for national certification, they must maintain their certification. Completion of specified continuing education hours to continue to develop and expand skills is one of the major requirements for certification maintenance. Continuing education contact hours confer credit for participating in educational programs that update and develop professionals' skills.

Another requirement to maintain national certifications is the adherence to NBCC's *Code of Ethics*. Each year, with the submission of the *NBCC Statement of Annual Maintenance Fees*, certificants are reminded that they must disclose within sixty days any legal or criminal complaints or actions. Additionally, the NBCC ethics office reviews concerns submitted by clients, members of the public or other professionals. All disclosures and charges are processed according to the policies described in the NBCC *Ethics Case Procedures.*

NBCC'S ACCREDITATION

As a method of quality assurance, NBCC voluntarily submits to a review of its certification processes. This helps assure counselors, legislators and other members of the public that national certification through NBCC meets standards consistent with professional credentialing organizations. In October 1985, NBCC was accredited by the National Commission for Certifying Agencies (NCCA). NCCA is an independent national regulatory organization that monitors the credentialing processes of its member agencies. Accreditation by the commission represents the foremost organizational recognition in national certification. Currently, the NCC and MAC are accredited by NCCA.

OTHER BENEFITS

Besides the most visible benefit of possession of quality certification by NBCC, the credential designation (e.g., NCC), there are many other benefits provided by national certification through NBCC.

Advocacy: In addition to supporting counselor licensure efforts, NBCC advocates for important changes relevant to professional counseling.

Professional distinction: Completion of a voluntary certification process demonstrates strong professional identity and a commitment to continued skill development.

Transferability: National certifications are not specific to certain states. This aids in the provision of referrals.

Low-cost liability insurance: NBCC offers, through Lockton Affinity, very reasonably priced insurance that is available to graduate students and certificants.

Access to discounted testing instruments: NBCC collaborates with the Institute for Personality and Ability Testing, Inc. (IPAT) to allow certificants access to quality testing instruments at reduced costs.

Discounted subscriptions to Psychology Today: NBCC partners with *Psychology Today* to allow certificants access to discounted subscriptions to the popular magazine. There is also a method for certificants to earn continuing education credits.

Access to quality research: NBCC's new academic journal, *The Professional Counselor,* is an online resource for counselors, counselor educators, graduate students and members of the public.

AFFILIATES

As an organization which continues to grow, NBCC maintains a strong, reliable reputation for providing quality counseling certifications, and other organizations have sought information about how to create similar processes. As a result, NBCC has created a separate organization, the Center for Credentialing and Education (CCE). CCE offers services in association and credential management, credential review and exam administration. CCE has also developed or is in the process of developing other credentials in human services, clinical supervision, career facilitation, correctional training, distance counseling, distance facilitation and coaching.

Many counseling leaders in other countries studied in the United States and pursued national certification through NBCC because no formal regulation or recognition systems existed in their home countries. As more professionals returned to their home countries and NBCC travels abroad increased, board and staff members were increasingly being approached about collaboration in professionalization mechanisms. NBCC responded by creating a division, NBCC International (NBCC-I), to promote the strengthening of the counseling profession worldwide. NBCC-I works collaboratively with other countries' leaders and counseling experts to meet local needs. The projects are always locally determined with organizational collaboration provided by NBCC-I. Projects range from the creation of certification systems to the formation of response mechanisms, such as the Mental Health Facilitator (MHF) program. This program helps increase access to mental health services especially in remote areas and in underserved populations.

Promoting access to those in remote and underserved areas is not limited to other countries. Recently, economic and military events have led to an increase in need. Another related organization, the NBCC Foundation, responded by creating scholarship opportunities for those who are interested in counseling careers and desire to serve either the military population or those in rural, underserved areas. The NBCC Foundation continues to be dedicated to promoting mental health through the advancement of professional counseling and credentialing.

REFERENCES

American Educational Research Association, American Psychological Association, and National Council on Measurement in Education. (1999). *Standards for educational and psychological testing.* Washington, D.C.: American Educational Research Association.

Tyler, H.R., Moskow, M.H., Walsh, E.B., Hampton, R. E., & Flemming, A.E. (1978). *Section 63: Uniform guidelines on employee selection procedure; 43 FR 38295.* Retrieved from http://www.uniformguidelines.com/uniformguidelines.html

Chapter 8

Chi Sigma Iota
Counseling Academic and Professional Honor Society International

Thomas J. Sweeney
Chi Sigma Iota Executive Director

WHAT IS CHI SIGMA IOTA?

Chi Sigma Iota (CSI) is the international honor society of professional counseling. It was established in 1985 through the efforts of leaders whose desire was to provide recognition for outstanding achievement and service within the profession. CSI was created for counselors-in-training, counselor educators, and professional counselors whose career commitment is to personal and professional excellence.

Our Mission

Our mission is to promote scholarship, research, professionalism, leadership, advocacy, and excellence in counseling, and to recognize high attainment in the pursuit of academic clinical excellence in the profession of counseling. We promote a strong professional identity through members (professional counselors, counselor educators and students) who contribute to the realization of a healthy society by fostering wellness and human dignity.

Who Are Our Members?

Because common usage of the term *counselor* can be misleading, professional counselors are distinguished by their preparation at the graduate level in pursuit of both master's and doctoral degrees in counselor education. One's highest or terminal degree is evidence of a desire to identify with the profession. Membership supports the mission of the society.

For purposes of clarity among helping professionals who use counseling as a method or its techniques, the graduate education of members of the profession of counseling are defined by the national standards of the Council for Accreditation of Counseling and Related Educational Programs (CACREP). Individuals whose programs of study in counselor education are accredited by the Council of Rehabilitation Education (CORE) also are eligible for membership.

Promoting Excellence in Preparation and Practice

Academic excellence for individuals invited to membership is measured by grade point average (3.5 or better on a 4.0 system). In addition the individuals must be "...deemed promising for endorsement as a professional counselor whose ethical judgment and behavior will be exemplary" (*CSI Bylaws*, 2008, p. 2). Chapters may require more than a full academic term of study in counseling to make such a determination before endorsing new members. That said CSI strives to be proactive in encouraging diversity in leadership and deliberate in reaching out and extending the honor of membership to all who have excelled in their academics. Graduate school admission criteria usually mean that the "best and brightest" have been admitted. All should be capable of academic excellence and membership in CSI.

Chapters must be located in university or college programs preparing graduates eligible for credentialing as professional counselors. All must fundamentally meet the minimum standards as defined by CACREP. All new and renewing chapters must be nationally accredited within five years of activation. Most of our 270 plus chapters are already located in nationally accredited counselor education programs.

CSI has always required the National Certified Counselor credential (NCC), a professional counseling certification of the National Board for Certified Counselors, and/or state credentials for alumni and faculty being endorsed for membership through our chapters. Continuing education and adherence to our professional ethical codes are expectations for all members.

Worldwide Membership

CSI is growing steadily. We are honoring over 5,000 new members per year. Currently there are over 13,000 annual dues paying members and over 70,000 members overall. For the latter group, for a modest annual dues fee they can become active members. Over one half of the annual dues paying members are professional practitioners, counseling supervisors, and counselor educators. As a consequence CSI is one of the three largest professional counselors' organizations in the world.

Most members in other countries were educated in United States university programs. With professional counseling in other countries on the rise, we expect to support more chapters in more countries in the future. Our Philippines chapter, Iota Phi, celebrated its 20th anniversary in 2008.

ACTIVITIES AND ACCOMPLISHMENTS

Providing Recognition and Leaders for the Profession

- All members have been honored and recognized publicly for their excellence as students and practitioners of professional counseling.
- Leaders and scholars about whom the initiates have heard or read volunteer to speak at initiations all over the country *pro bono*.
- Leadership preparation is an integral and substantive part of all that CSI does as a co-curricular partner through our Chapter Faculty Advisors.
- In addition, CSI has endorsed three major works by CSI members including
  - Locke, D.C., Myers, J.E., & Herr, E.H. (Eds). (2001). *The handbook of counseling*. Riverside, CA: Sage Publications.
  - West, J.D., Osborn, C.J., & Bubenzer, D.L. (Eds). (2003). *Leaders and legacies: Contributions to the counseling profession*. Muncie, IN: Accelerated Development Inc., a Taylor & Francis Co.
  - Chang, C.Y., Barrio Minton, C., Dixon, A.L., Myers, J.E., & Sweeney, T.J. (Eds). (2011). *Professional counseling excellence through leadership and advocacy*. New York: Routledge, Taylor & Francis Group.
- Chapters have received over $660,000 directly from CSI to support leadership preparation, advocacy, and many other activities.
- Awards of $160,000 in fellowships and internships have been given to individuals to attend CSI day leadership preparation and to participate in year round activities of the society.

- As a consequence, CSI is unique in contributing directly to the counselor education programs of which they are a part to develop leaders and promote a clear and resilient professional identity.
- Notably, every organization listed in *Counseling Today*, the newsletter for the American Counseling Association (ACA), has CSI members in its leadership.

Collaborating to Promote Excellence

Through the work of countless volunteers, CSI has been at the forefront of efforts to promote excellence in the profession and to advocate for the place of counseling among service providers. These efforts include

- Co-publishing and distributing a professional pamphlet on "Client Rights and Responsibilities" with NBCC, making donations to the ACA for its library to improve services to its members, donating funds to support an ACA Professionalization Conference, and continuing to support both ACA and the Association for Counselor Education and Supervision (ACES) conferences and membership.
- Sponsoring two national Counselor Advocacy Leadership conferences with representatives from associations, credentialing and accreditation bodies.

Organizational Example and Excellence

Reprints of articles and citations in refereed journals are testimony to the value of our chief publication, the *Exemplar*. Our Web site (www.csi-net.org) is a rich resource of materials, information and news and has been cited for its excellence. As members of the Association of College Honor Societies (ACHS), we are required to periodically demonstrate organizational excellence through compliance with its high standards for member organizations, much like accreditation organizations.

FUTURE VISION

Chi Sigma Iota is a dynamic blend of new aspiring leaders and those whose experience, knowledge and generosity support a clear and unequivocal mission. Our growth in members and chapters is steady. Leadership development of members and support for our chapters will be ever increasing. Advocacy for the profession and social justice for those we serve will be the substance around which leadership will be focused. Our earnest efforts to encourage counselors in other countries will be through networking that supports their priorities and culture. We aspire to do all that we can for our members and the profession but to do so within our means such that is it accomplished well. As a consequence we will continue to collaborate, support and promote the missions of the counseling organizations and agencies upon whom we all depend.

For further information:

Chi Sigma Iota
P.O. Box 35448
Greensboro, NC 27425-5448
Phone/Fax: (336) 841-8180
Web site: www.csi-net.org
Email: info@csi-net.org

REFERENCES

Chi Sigma Iota Bylaws. (2008). Article 4. p. 2. Retrieved from http://www.csi-net.org/associations/2151/files/CSI_Bylaws.pdf

Counselor Preparation Programs

Chapter 9

Entry-Level Counselor Preparation Programs
Master's Degrees

Professional counselors-in-training pursue a master's degree with specialty study in an identified area. Most often students in counselor preparation programs focus on the core areas of human growth and development, assessment, group work, helping relationships, career development, research and program evaluation, professional orientation and ethical practice, and social and cultural diversity. Besides these foundation courses, students take courses specific to their specialty area and participate in supervised clinical experiences appropriate to their intended areas of practice. CACREP's Web site (http://www.cacrep.org) outlines CACREP standards for the scope of these academic and clinical experiences.

PROGRAMS OFFERED

Information was collected from 210 master's programs that responded to the Data Collection Form. Programs indicated which specialty areas were offered by their institutions. According to these data, the specialty areas of community, with 41 programs, and school counseling, with 70 programs, were by far those most commonly identified. These two areas constituted 53 percent of all entry-level programs offered.

ADMISSIONS AND GRADUATES

The number of students admitted to entry-level counseling programs range from a high of 150 and a low of 3 with an average admission group of 23.

TABLE 9.1 Number of Students Admitted
and Graduated Yearly in Entry Level Counseling Programs

	Number of Programs Responding	High	Low	Average	SD
Admitted yearly	184	150	3	23	19.6
Graduated yearly	179	70	0	18	13.5
Female	139	175	0	29	30.8
Male	138	40	0	9	8.9
Average age	82	42	23	29	4.2

Some programs have as many as 70 graduates per year, and others have as few as zero. The average number of graduates is 18 per year. The majority of students are female and students range in age from 23 to 42. Most master's level counseling students enroll in and graduate from community counseling or school counseling programs. Table 9.1 shows the average number of students admitted and graduated yearly for counseling preparation programs that reported this information.

ADMISSION REQUIREMENTS

Counselor preparation programs require a variety of information before admitting students. Standardized tests such as the Graduate Record Examination (GRE) and the Miller Analogies Test (MAT) are used by some programs as a part of their admission requirements. Of the 144 programs that responded to this portion of the survey, 78 programs, or 54% of the respondents, require the GRE. Some respondents, 33 or 25%, require the MAT. The majority of programs (99%) require a degree for admission to the counselor preparation program. Programs also reported the average grade point average (GPA) of students admitted. Among responding institutions, the average GPA was 2.91. Some programs ask applicants to have work experience, to submit recommendation letters, or to participate in an interview before they are admitted to the counselor preparation program. Of the programs that responded to this section of the survey, 34 required work experiences, 176 asked for letters of recommendation, and 138 interviewed applicants. Table 9.2 summarizes requirements for admission to entry-level counselor preparation programs.

GRADUATION REQUIREMENTS

Students in counselor preparation programs complete supervised practicum and internship hours before graduation. Program requirements may vary according to specialty areas. According to CACREP standards, practicum in

TABLE 9.2 Admission Requirements
for Entry Level Counseling Programs

	Number of Programs Responding	High	Low	Average	SD	Yes	No	% Yes
GRE required	144					78	66	54%
MAT required	132					33	99	25%
Degree required	144					142	2	99%
Interview	171					138	33	81%
GPA	159	3.25	2.5	2.91	0.17			
Work experience	34	3	0	0.91	0.83			
Recommendation letters	176	5	2	2.84	0.56			

GRE: Graduate Record Examination; *MAT:* Miller Analogies Test; *GPA:* Grade Point Average

entry-level programs includes 100 clock hours, with 40 or more of those hours in direct service. CACREP standards define a minimum of 600 clock hours for internship, with 240 or more of those involving direct service. Practicum and internship also involve group supervision of one and one-half hours per week and individual supervision of one hour per week. Responding programs required an average of 139 practicum hours and 596 internship hours. Table 9.3 contains information about practicum and internship requirements.

Successful completion of coursework is a standard requirement for graduation. Of the programs that responded to this portion of the Data Collection Form, most operate on semester systems. These programs required an average of 53 semester hours for graduation. The 13 programs that reported operating on a quarter system required an average of 75 quarter hours for graduation. Further information on academic hour requirements is contained in Table 9.3.

Programs may have other graduation requirements, including a thesis, comprehensive examination, oral examination and/or portfolio. According to the data collected, 9 require a thesis, 133 require a comprehensive examination, 21 require an oral exam, and 59 require portfolios. Table 9.4 details these additional graduation requirements from responding programs.

TABLE 9.3 Graduation Requirements
for Master's Degrees in Counseling

	Number of Programs Responding	High	Low	Average	SD
Practicum hours	181	1000	32	139	115
Internship hours	176	900	150	596	116
Semester hours	181	92	15	53	9
Quarter hours	13	92	41	75	13

TABLE 9.4 Graduation Requirements for Master's
Degrees in Counseling: Other Requirements

	Number of Programs Responding	Yes	No	% Yes
Thesis	146	9	137	6%
Comprehensive exam	173	133	40	77%
Oral exam	125	21	104	17%
Portfolio	136	59	77	43%

JOB SETTINGS AFTER GRADUATION

Most graduates of counselor preparation programs find employment in settings related to their specialty areas, according to the survey data. Thirty-five percent of master graduates work in agencies and forty-one percent work in schools. Table 9.5 details graduates' job settings the first year after completing entry-level programs. Some graduates choose to pursue an advanced degree after finishing the entry-level program. Chapter 11 contains information about doctoral level preparation programs.

TABLE 9.5 Job Settings After Graduation

Setting	Number of Programs Responding	Percent of Graduates
Advanced education	134	6%
Agency	118	35%
Assisted living facilities	8	5%
Counselor education	80	1%
Churches	16	9%
Church ministry	5	3%
Corporate settings	10	6%
Criminal justice settings	17	10%
Government	14	8%
Higher education staff	98	13%
Hospice	11	6%
Hospitals	30	18%
Other	104	12%
Private practice	104	6%
School—elementary	103	13%
School—middle	105	11%
School—secondary	108	17%
Teaching	24	14%
Working with developmentally disabled	19	11%

Chapter 10

Specialist Counselor Preparation Programs

Some students may choose to pursue an educational specialist degree in counseling. These programs may build upon the foundations of the entry-level program and may allow their graduates access to advanced certification.

PROGRAMS OFFERED

Information was collected from 27 programs through the Data Collection Form. According to these data, school counseling, with 6 programs, and community counseling, with 4, are the most commonly identified specialist areas. These two areas constituted 38 percent of all specialist programs offered.

ADMISSIONS AND GRADUATES

Specialist programs enroll and graduate fewer students than entry-level programs. The number of students admitted yearly for a specialist's degree ranges from 2 to 40 students. The number of students who graduate from specialist programs ranges from 1 to 28 per year. Females outnumber males and the average age of students is 33 years. Table 10.1 contains the average number of students admitted and graduated annually from different counseling preparation programs that reported this information.

TABLE 10.1 Number of Students Admitted and Graduated
Yearly in Specialist Counseling Programs

	Number of Programs Responding	High	Low	Average	SD
Admitted yearly	25	40	2	11	8.4
Graduated yearly	25	28	1	8	6.4
Female	18	75	2	18	17.8
Male	16	25	1	7	7.7
Average age	5	44	27	33	6.5

ADMISSION REQUIREMENTS

Specialist counselor preparation programs require a variety of information before admitting students. Some use standardized tests such as the Graduate Record Examination (GRE) and the Miller Analogies Test (MAT) as a part of their admission requirements. Programs also reported the average grade point average (GPA) of students admitted. Of the programs that responded, 10 require the GRE (71%) and five require the MAT (38%). Across all programs, the GPA average is a 3.07. Table 10.2 contains information related to the specialty programs' requirements.

Some programs ask applicants to have a master's degree, have work experience, to submit recommendation letters, and/or to participate in an interview. Of the programs that responded, 12 required a master's degree, and seven held interviews for applicants to their programs. In addition, three programs required work experience, and 22 required letters of recommendation. Table 10.2 contains information specific to specialty programs.

TABLE 10.2 Admission Requirements
for Specialist Counseling Programs

	Number of Programs Responding	High	Low	Average	SD	Yes	No	% Yes
GRE required	14					10	4	71%
MAT required	13					5	8	38%
Interview	13					7	6	54%
Master's required	13					12	1	92%
GPA	7	3.5	3	3.07	0.19			
Work experience	3	2	2	2.00	0			
Recommendation letters	22	3	2	2.91	0.29			

GRE: Graduate Record Examination; *MAT:* Miller Analogies Test; *GPA:* Grade Point Average

TABLE 10.3 Graduation Requirements for Specialist
Counseling Programs

	Number of Programs Responding	High	Low	Average	SD
Practicum hours	8	120	100	113	10.4
Internship hours	18	900	150	524	205.3

TABLE 10.4 Graduation Requirements for Specialist
Degrees in Counseling: Other Requirements

	Number of Programs Responding	Yes	No	% Yes
Thesis	17	4	13	24%
Comprehensive exam	25	20	5	80%
Oral exam	12	2	10	17%
Portfolio	11	3	8	27%

GRADUATION REQUIREMENTS

Students in specialist counselor preparation programs must complete supervised practicum and internship hours before graduation. Required hours may vary according to specialty area. Among the eight programs providing information on practicum hours, the average number required was 113. The average number of internship hours was 524 among the 18 programs that responded. Table 10.3 contains information related to required practicum and internship hours.

Successful completion of coursework is a standard requirement for graduation from a specialist counselor preparation program. The average number of graduate hours required for the specialist programs that responded to this portion of the Data Collection Form was 39.7 semester hours.

Programs may have exit requirements other than course completion. Examples of some other graduation requirements are writing a thesis, passing a comprehensive or oral examination, or compiling a portfolio. Four specialist programs reported requiring a thesis, 20 require comprehensive examinations, 2 have oral examinations and 3 require a portfolio. These data and the number of programs that answered this portion of the Data Collection Form are presented in Table 10.4.

JOB SETTINGS AFTER GRADUATION

Graduates' work opportunities after completing a specialist counselor education program mirror many of those of entry-level practitioners. Table 10.5 lists percentages of graduates by job setting after graduation.

TABLE 10.5 Job Settings After Graduation

Setting	Number of Programs Responding	Percent of Graduates
Advanced education	17	9%
Agency	16	36%
Counselor education	0	0%
Higher education staff	7	2%
Managed care	7	1%
Other	10	14%
Private practice	9	7%
School—elementary	14	10%
School—middle	14	9%
School—secondary	14	11%

Chapter 11

Doctoral-Level Counselor Preparation Programs

Professional counselors also may choose to pursue a doctoral degree. Doctoral programs build upon the foundations of the entry-level programs. CACREP accredits doctoral-level counselor education and supervision programs but does not differentiate among specialty areas at the doctoral level. To review CACREP standards for the scope and type of academic and clinical experience for doctoral level programs, visit http://www.cacrep.org.

PROGRAMS OFFERED

Forty-one programs responded to questions about doctoral-level programs on the Data Collection Form. Programs indicated which specialty areas were offered by their institutions. According to these data, the specialty area of counselor education was the most commonly identified with 20 programs. Counselor education programs constituted 49 percent of all doctoral programs offered.

ADMISSIONS AND GRADUATES

Doctoral-level programs enroll and graduate fewer students than entry-level programs. Programs reported admitting an average of four to five students per year to advanced degree programs. The number of graduates from doctoral programs ranges from none to 12 per year. More females graduated and the average age of a doctoral graduate was 34. Table 11.1 contains the average number of students admitted and graduated annually for advanced counselor preparation programs that reported this information.

TABLE 11.1   Number of Students Admitted and Graduated Yearly in Doctoral Level Programs

	Number of Programs Responding	High	Low	Average	SD
Admitted yearly	33	14	0	5	4.1
Graduated yearly	30	12	0	4	3.5
Female	18	45	2	12	13.5
Male	17	15	1	4	3.9
Average age	8	46	25	34	6.8

ADMISSION REQUIREMENTS

Doctoral-level counselor preparation programs require a variety of information before admitting students. Some use standardized tests such as the Graduate Record Examination (GRE) and the Miller Analogies Test (MAT) as a part of their admission requirements. Of the 41 programs that responded to this part of the survey, 24 or 73% require the GRE and two or 10% require the MAT. Programs also reported an average grade point average (GPA) of 3.41 for students admitted. Thirty-two programs required a master's degree. Table 11.2 contains this information.

Some programs ask applicants to have work experience, to submit recommendation letters, and/or to participate in an interview. Of those that responded, 17 programs reported requiring work experiences, 35 asked for letters of recommendation, and 33 held interviews for applicants to their programs. Table 11.2 contains more admission information.

TABLE 11.2   Admission Requirements for Doctoral Level Counseling Programs

	Number of Programs Responding	High	Low	Average	SD	Yes	No	% Yes
GRE required	33					24	9	73%
MAT required	20					2	18	10%
Master's required	35					32	3	91%
Interview	35					33	2	94%
GPA	30	4.0	3.0	3.41	0.48			
Work experience	17	3	0	1.82	0.64			
Recommendation letters	35	4	2	2.80	0.47			

GRE: Graduate Record Examination; *MAT:* Miller Analogies Test; *GPA:* Grade Point Average

GRADUATION REQUIREMENTS

Students in doctoral-level counselor preparation programs complete supervised practicum and internship hours before graduation. These hours may vary according to the specialty area of the doctoral program. Information provided on the Data Collection Form indicated an average of 213 practicum hours required in the 21 programs that responded, and 641 internship hours required in the 34 programs that responded. Table 11.3 contains information related to required practicum and internship hours.

Successful completion of coursework is also a standard requirement for graduation. The average number of graduate hours required for the doctoral-level programs that responded to this portion of the Data Collection Form was 89 semester hours with a range from 60 to 120. The average across the three programs reporting quarter hours was 110, with a range from 90 to 150. Table 11.3 also contains information on this.

Programs may have additional exit requirements. Examples of other graduation requirements include writing a thesis or dissertation, passing a comprehensive examination or oral examination, and/or compiling a portfolio. According to the data collected from 36 programs, all reported requiring a thesis or dissertation. Thirty-three of 35 responding reported requiring a comprehensive examination, 23 of 25 required oral examinations, and 2 of 7 responding include portfolios as part of their graduation requirements. Table 11.4 details the additional graduation requirements for the doctoral programs that answered this portion of the Data Collection Form.

TABLE 11.3 Graduation Requirements for Doctoral Degrees

	Number of Programs Responding	High	Low	Average	SD
Practicum hours	21	1270	50	213	313
Internship hours	34	2000	160	641	279
Semester hours	32	120	60	89	16
Quarter hours	3	150	90	110	35

TABLE 11.4 Graduation Requirements for Doctoral Degrees in Counseling: Other Requirements

	Number of Programs Responding	Yes	No	% Yes
Thesis/dissertation	36	36	0	100%
Comprehensive exam	35	33	2	94%
Oral exam	25	23	2	92%
Portfolio	7	2	5	29%

TABLE 11.5 Job Settings After Graduation

Setting	Number of Programs Responding	Percent of Graduates
Advanced education	24	12%
Agency	27	12%
Counselor education	20	18%
Higher education	23	15%
Managed care	18	5%
Other	19	17%
Private practice	26	10%
School—elementary	14	1%
School—middle	17	5%
School—secondary	20	5%

JOB SETTINGS AFTER GRADUATION

According to information reported on the Data Collection Form, the highest percentage of graduates goes on to jobs in counselor education. Table 11.5 details percentages of graduates by job setting the first year after completing a doctoral-level program.

Chapter 12

Issues and Needs of International Students in Counselor Preparation Programs
A Literature Review

Kok-Mun Ng and Jared Lau
The University of North Carolina at Charlotte

Counselor preparation programs have played a major role in contributing to the growth of the counseling profession in the United States by producing practitioners, supervisors, educators, and leaders in the field across the globe, and the counseling profession has now expanded rapidly beyond the U.S. to other parts of the world (Heppner, Leong, & Gerstein, 2008). Many professional counselors and counselor educators around the world were either trained in the U.S. or trained by native trainers who were graduates of American counselor preparation programs (Leung et al., 2009). As such, it could be said that international counseling students (ICSs) trained in American counselor preparation programs have played and continue to play a significant role in the development of the counseling profession across the globe. Interestingly, only in the last 10 years has the literature begun to address the specific issues and needs of international students in counselor preparation programs and related helping professions such as applied psychology and marriage and family therapy (e.g., Killian, 2001; Morris & Lee, 2004; Ng, 2006a, 2006b; Ng & Smith, 2009; Nilsson & Anderson, 2004; Pattison, 2003; Smith & Ng, 2009).

In this chapter we will present a thematic review of the counseling literature on ICSs. Literature from other helping professions such as applied psychology and marriage and family therapy also will be referenced whenever relevant. We will summarize and discuss the enrollment information on ICSs presented in the present volume of *Counselor Preparation*. Because of page limitation we will not critique methodological issues in the research on ICSs. We will conclude the chapter with a summary of recommendations for training and supervising ICSs.

ENROLLMENT REPRESENTATION

The enrollment of international students in the U.S. and other developed countries has been on the rise in the last several decades (Haigh, 2002; Institute of International Education [IIE], 2009). Enrollment statistics on ICSs in graduate counselor training programs had not been reported in the literature until recently when Ng (2006b) surveyed the presence of international students in American counselor preparation programs that were accredited by the Council for Accreditation of Counseling and Related Educational Programs (CACREP) in 2004. Ng's findings revealed that at least 41% of the accredited programs at the time had international students enrolled in them and close to 50% of programs had had international students in the preceding three years. Based on the number provided by the responding programs, ICSs constituted about 3% of enrollment, a percentage reflective of the enrollment of international students in the education field at the time (IIE, 2004). But Ng's study was limited to CACREP programs. The representation of ICSs in non-CACREP programs and non-American programs remains unknown though ICSs are studying in various countries such as Malaysia, Mexico, Turkey, Australia and the United Kingdom.

It was decided that enrollment information on international students should be gathered for the present edition of *Counselor Preparation*. To gather this information, programs were asked if (a) international students were currently enrolled in their programs, and (b) if yes, how many? Of the 116 programs that participated in the study, 70 (68.3%) reported having international students currently enrolled, 28 (24.1%) reported having no ICSs currently enrolled, and 18 (15.5%) did not respond to this question.

Of the 70 programs that reported having ICSs currently enrolled, 55 (78.6%) programs provided information on the number of ICSs enrolled. The number of ICSs in these 55 programs totaled 276, making an average of 5.02 ICSs per program. These numbers should be viewed with caution because the number of enrolled ICSs ranged from 1 to 30. Nine programs reported having one ICS enrolled, 18 reported 2, 4 reported 3, 5 programs reported 4, 12 reported 5, 1 reported 8, 1 reported 10, 1 reported 12, 2 reported 20, and 2 reported 30. To gain a global picture of the representation of international counseling students more information is needed, such as number, country of origin and training specialty. Based on the statistics, it seems reasonable to conclude that although the number of international students per program is low, their presence in U.S. counseling training programs is not insignificant.

ACADEMIC AND PSYCHOSOCIAL CHALLENGES

Challenges confronting international students studying in American and other Western higher education have been well-researched and discussed in the literature (see Chen, 1999; Yoon & Portman, 2004). Common stressors international students tend to encounter are (a) second language anxiety, (b) educational stressors (e.g., performance expectations, system adjustment stress, test-taking anxiety), (c) social stressors (e.g., culture shock, social isolation, financial concerns, racial discrimination), and (d) legal stressors (e.g., keeping a required number of credit hours to maintain legal status) (Chen, 1999; Paige, 1990). Some of these stressors are in addition to those commonly experienced by domestic students. Because of their unfamiliarity with American teaching methodologies and American students' studying and learning styles, as well as their foreign English accents, some international students who work as graduate teaching assistants also encounter challenges their domestic counterparts do not (Mori, 2000).

The above-mentioned stressors seem to be common among ICSs as well. Compared to domestic counseling students, ICSs attending American counselor preparation programs reported experiencing higher levels of academic problems, English proficiency problems, cultural adjustment issues, and discrimination by faculty members and fellow students (Ng & Smith, 2009). American counselor educators who had trained ICSs also noted similar challenges confronting these students (Ng, 2006a). Counselor educators in Ng's study further reported that ICSs from non-Western countries tended to face greater difficulties in these areas than their counterparts from Western countries. In addition, international students who were more successful tended to experience these challenges less than those who were less successful. International students in American marriage and family therapy programs had also been reported to experience similar challenges such as language difficulties, cultural adjustment challenges, pressure to assimilate American norms and values, and the need to acclimatize to an American training context and approach (Killian, 2001; Mittal & Wieling, 2006).

A qualitative research study conducted by Pattison (2003) revealed that ICSs' training experiences could be related to cultural differences in teaching and learning styles. For example, Southeast Asian students prefer the familiarity of didactic teaching methods, whereas African students enjoy lively discussion. Also, African students tend to share feelings openly compared to Chinese students who tend to be more reserved emotionally. Having to adjust to the teaching styles of the instructors in the host country and navigate through the learning style differences among fellow students could be a source of stress to some ICSs (Pattison, 2003).

Besides the difficulties related to pedagogy and learning style differences, some ICSs may also have to deal with learning content that conflicts with their cultural beliefs and values. For example, some students may experience person-centered counseling to be focusing on the exploration of feelings, an emphasis that goes contrary to their cultural value that downplays emotions (Pattison, 2003). Ng's (2006a) study further reveals that non-Western ICSs tended to experience more conflicts with Western understanding of and approaches to treating mental health compared to ICSs from Western countries and American domestic counseling students.

A related academic issue that has been preliminarily explored concerns ICSs' experiences and perceptions of their training in multicultural counseling competencies (Smith & Ng, 2009). Though international students in Smith and Ng's study reported that they perceived their multicultural counseling training to be rather useful in assisting them in gaining multicultural knowledge and awareness, they experienced this training as less useful in helping them acquire multicultural counseling skills. Also, findings in the Smith and Ng study reveal dissatisfaction among some ICSs with the multicultural counseling training they received and indicate limited applicability of what was taught to their country of origin. It seems, therefore, that ICSs need to spend extra effort to critically examine and digest what they have learned so they can apply their learning appropriately when they return to work in their native countries. This is particularly critical when they want to avoid propagating a Western/American approach of counseling.

The literature has also shed light on the career-related difficulties and dilemmas ICSs face. Some of these students may require more academic and career support (Mittal & Weiling, 2006) because of their unfamiliarity with counseling training and related employment options in the U.S. and their native countries (Ng & Smith, 2009). Because counseling is not yet a developed profession in most countries outside of North America, finding a counseling job will be a serious challenge when students return to their native countries upon graduation.

Though there is much literature on the mental health needs of international students and treatment issues for this population (e.g., Singaravelu & Pope, 2006), studies focusing on the mental health issues of ICSs remain unavailable. Ng and Smith's (2009) exploratory findings indicate that international students and domestic students in American counselor preparation programs do not differ significantly in their experience of mental or emotional distress. ICSs from non-Western countries who were less successful, however, were noted by their professors to experience more mental or emotional distress than students from non-Western countries who were more successful (Ng, 2006a). It seems that international students who were not doing well in their training compared to those who were doing well tended to experience more psychosocial and academically related difficulties. A similar trend was observed among American counseling students (Ng, 2006a).

CLINICAL TRAINING AND SUPERVISORY CHALLENGES

Unlike many fields of study, clinical training and supervision are major curricular components in counseling and related helping fields. Counseling also relies heavily on verbal communication and proficiency and cultural competence when providing direct services to clients. Besides impacting students' academic performance, linguistic challenges also affect ICSs' clinical training and supervisory experience. Language barriers can affect their communication with their clients (Ng & Smith, 2009). ICSs whose English accents are different from their American clients may be perceived by their clients who are less multiculturally aware and appreciative of differences as less expert, less trustworthy, and less attractive than counselors who speak with a "standard" accent (Fuertes, Potere, & Ramirez, 2002). They may also experience overt and covert racist and discriminatory attitudes from clients (Killian, 2001; Mittal & Wieling, 2006). Some ICSs may experience difficulties understanding the cultural contexts of their clients (Mittal & Wieling, 2006). It seems reasonable to perceive the difficulties ICSs experience in clinical courses and the difficulties fitting into their clinical placements (Ng, 2006a) as related to their language proficiency, racial heritage and nationality, and acculturation process. Their foreign accent and unfamiliarity with the American educational system and learning styles may also negatively affect the respect, trust, and acceptance from students they teach or supervise (Pedersen, 1991).

Though Nilsson and Anderson's (2004) findings are based on international doctoral students in professional psychology programs accredited by the American Psychological Association, we believe that they apply to international students in counselor preparation programs. Nilsson and Anderson found that international doctoral trainees who were less acculturated to the American culture reported less counseling skill self-efficacy, a weaker supervisory working alliance, greater role ambiguity in supervision, and more discussion of cultural issues in supervision. Nilsson and Anderson further noted that a positive supervisory working alliance allowed international students to address their cultural concerns, learn about the U.S. culture, and obtain support and guidance on how to work with cultural issues in therapy and supervision.

A perceived lack of multicultural competence of their supervisors has also been found to be a challenge for international trainees (Mori, Inman, & Caskie, 2009). Some ICSs may encounter difficulties with clinical supervisors who are culturally insensitive to the learning and communication differences of international students. It would be difficult for ICSs who subscribe to a strong cultural proscription against "talking back" to authority figures to respond when they encounter hostility from faculty members or site supervisors (Killian, 2001; Mittal & Wieling, 2006). Such encounters become a relational stressor to these students. Both Mori et al.'s and Nilsson and Dodds' (2006) studies indicate that international trainees experience higher levels of satisfaction when they are engaged in higher levels of cultural discussion with their supervisors. It has been argued that trainees need to trust their supervisors and experience them as knowledgeable before they feel comfortable to bring up their concerns related to culture, language barriers, and so forth (Killian, 2001; Nilsson, 2007).

CONTRIBUTIONS AND STRENGTHS

International students have been recognized as one of the most important resources for achieving internationalization in higher education, campus diversity, and promoting a multicultural learning environment, besides the economic gains international student enrollment brings to the host countries (Peterson, Briggs, Dreasher, Horner, & Nelson, 1999). Exploratory studies on ICSs reveal that their participation in counseling and related training programs contributed to their trainers, fellow trainees, and clients (Killian, 2001; Ng, 2006a). When compared to domestic counseling students, ICSs shared a strong belief that they had much to contribute to the learning environment of their training programs (Ng & Smith, 2009). This indicates that ICSs do recognize what they can bring to their learning environment. Existing studies have not explored the specific nature of the contributions, however. It is our belief that the presence of ICSs is likely to have the following potential impacts:

1. International students bring their cultural viewpoints to class discussions, interactions, and assignments that help to expand the scope of the discourse of theory and practice of counseling and supervision.
2. Out-of-class interactions with international students provide domestic students, faculty, and supervisors opportunities to gain cross-cultural knowledge, awareness, and skills.
3. The cultural and learning style differences of international students force counselor educators and supervisors to expand (a) their culturally encapsulated view on multiculturalism and diversity to include a more global perspective and (b) the learning content and teaching methods to meet the needs of all students, including international students. In so doing, internationalization of counselor training will be achieved.

ICSs have and will continue to play a major role in facilitating the process of internationalization of the counseling profession because they bring their training back to their home countries after graduation (Leung et al., 2009).

Many of these international counseling graduates are instrumental in establishing professional counseling associations, counselor preparation programs, counseling licensure, and so forth across the globe. International counseling graduates who decided to stay in the U.S. and other host countries also contribute to the profession through teaching, research, practice, and other professional and community services. Many of them bring an international flavor and perspective to their work.

RECOMMENDATIONS FOR TRAINEES AND SUPERVISORS

Based on findings in the literature and our personal experiences working with ICSs, we provide the following training and supervision recommendations for working with ICSs. These recommendations are provided as a starting point for trainees and supervisors who are involved in training ICSs. We encourage readers to modify these recommendations based on the specific and unique needs of the students, location and setting of training site, and graduate training program capabilities. Our recommendations are categorized into two main themes: cross-cultural supervision and training and student mentoring.

Cross-Cultural Supervision and Training

Understanding and knowledge of cultural traditions, beliefs, values, and non-verbal norms play an integral role in the development of the therapeutic relationship and empathy with clients' feelings and experiences (Gutierrez, 1982). As such, supervisors can assist ICSs in developing these skills by openly discussing and exploring the impact of culture on clinical work and also exploring roles of the supervisee and supervisor in clinical supervision. As supervisees may be hesitant to bring up cultural concerns to their clinical supervisors, Nilsson and Anderson (2004) suggest that supervisors should take responsibility for broaching cultural topics in supervision.

In order to supervise ICSs effectively and help them to gain multicultural counseling competence, supervisors must possess this competence themselves. Culturally competent supervisors are knowledgeable about the cultural background of their international trainees, aware of their own biases and prejudices against international students, and skillful in fostering a positive cross-cultural supervisory working alliance and providing culturally sensitive training and supervision.

Supervisees who trust their supervisors and experience them as cross-culturally and multiculturally knowledgeable may feel more comfortable bringing up their concerns, including those related to culture and language barriers (Nilsson, 2007). A strong supervisory working alliance helps ICSs manage possible cultural and language barriers in supervision (Nilsson &

Anderson, 2004) and will also facilitate the development of clinical skills in ICSs. Engaging in multicultural discussions with ICSs can help to promote dialogue between supervisee and supervisor, and such dialogue can assert a positive impact on the supervisory working alliance and help increase ICSs' counseling self-efficacy. ICSs also can learn how to engage clients in cultural discussions when their supervisors model this behavior during supervision.

Given the unique cultural backgrounds and values of ICSs, we encourage supervisors to be flexible when working with ICSs regarding issues unique to their cultural backgrounds. For example, specific religious and cultural holidays of ICSs may pose scheduling conflicts with training and supervision. Being mindful of such culture-specific events, supervisors can discuss with their supervisees strategies on how to schedule supervision sessions to accommodate such events. For example, with Muslim students, supervisors might want to discuss client and supervision scheduling during Ramadan and other needs or accommodations their students may request to assist them through this time of fasting.

A common misconception about international students is that many already possess an advanced proficiency of the English language. However, gaining mastery of a new language requires a strenuous effort and substantial length of time (Takahashi, 1989) which many international students do not have, particularly when most ICSs are limited in their length of stay in the United States and will return to their home countries upon graduation. Therefore, supervisors should be mindful of language barriers and the potential for linguistic and cultural misunderstandings of their ICSs both in supervision and while working with clients. Supervisors may want to refrain from speaking in colloquialisms or speaking at a rapid pace while conversing with ICSs who have language proficiency challenges. Supervisors should also make a concerted effort to be mindful of the nonverbal cues that may suggest confusion or misunderstandings within ICSs and "check in" with ICSs for any potential misunderstandings. By checking in, supervisors can also serve as advocates and provide support to their ICSs in times of cultural and linguistic misunderstandings.

Supervisors also can be supportive of their ICSs by being mindful of extracurricular challenges faced by ICSs from institutional and governmental levels, such as financial stress and stress related to strict federal regulations surrounding international students' ability to work for pay. Supervisors can be mindful of the burdens placed on ICSs and offer their assistance in locating university funding, keep course assignments and deadlines flexible, and advocate for a manageable client caseload and schedule.

Due to the unique need of some ICSs to return to practice counseling in a social setting different from the United States, it has been suggested that ICSs should develop an individualized program of study that would allow them to gain knowledge, awareness, and skills pertinent to their own country and culture which are above and beyond what they would learn in an American training program (Ng, 2006a; Smith & Ng, 2009). Counselor educators and supervisors can assist their international students with developing personalized and contextualized course assignments, electives, clinical experiences, research projects, immersion experiences, and so forth that can challenge these students to personalize and contextualize their training. We believe that such an individualized learning experience will help ICSs be more prepared to apply the knowledge, awareness, skills and expertise they gain in the United States when they return home to work.

Student Mentoring

Student mentoring recently has grown in popularity in mental health professions (see, e.g., Wedding, McCartney, & Currey, 2009). Mentoring can take various forms. Wedding et al. suggest that mentoring can be as informal as serving as a confidant. Mentoring also can occur in more formal and intimate settings such as providing clinical supervision during internships. We believe that taking the time to invest in students not just as counselor trainees but also as unique individuals who bring unique worldviews, skills, and experiences can help promote the development of these students by validating them as valuable members of the learning community.

As international students are widely known to underutilize campus services such as counseling (Mori, 2000), counselor educators and supervisors can mentor their students by connecting them with resources to help enhance their academic and personal growth while attending school (e.g., international student services, counseling services, community organizations for specific cultural groups or nationalities). Trainers can also mentor ICSs by offering to collaborate on research projects relevant and unique to their interests and needs. The extra time involved in conducting research can be used both to get to know students on a more personal level and to mentor the students in the details and philosophy of conducting and publishing research.

As many ICSs choose to return to their home countries upon graduation, trainers can mentor their ICSs by helping them prepare for the re-entry process. For example, trainers, drawing on their own network, can connect international students with individuals in their respective home countries who may be able to help the students understand the local counseling employment situation. Trainers also can help ICSs research the procedures and requirements for obtaining local licensure and locating professional counseling organizations in their home countries. ICSs should be encouraged to take up leadership positions in counseling organizations in their home countries to promote counseling and advocate for mental health access particularly where professional counseling and mental health services are not well developed. Trainers can continue to offer support and guidance to students who have returned home on issues such as policy making and program design. Through continued consultation, collaboration on research and other scholarly activities, trainers will continue to play a role in advancing the profession of counseling across the globe.

CONCLUSION

Students from countries where counselor training is less developed will continue to enroll in counselor preparation programs in the United States and other countries that offer advanced training opportunities. The unique training and supervisory needs of these students should be taken into consideration by counselor educators and supervisors. This is particularly important because international counseling graduates have played and will continue to play a major role in the globalization of the counseling profession.

REFERENCES

Chen, C. P. (1999). Common stressors among international college students: Research and counseling implications. *Journal of College Counseling, 2*, 49–65.

Fuertes, J. N., Potere, J. C., & Ramirez, K. Y. (2002). Effects of speech accents on interpersonal evaluations: Implications for counseling. *Cultural Diversity and Ethnic Minority Psychology, 8*, 346–356.

Gutierrez, F. J. (1982). Working with minority counselor education students. *Counselor Education and Supervision, 21*(3), 218–226.

Haigh, M. J. (2002). Internationalisation of the curriculum: Designing inclusive education for a small world. *Journal of Geography in Higher Education, 26*(1), 49–66.

Heppner, P. P., Leong, F. T. L., & Gerstein, L. H. (2008). Counseling within a changing world: Meeting the psychological needs of societies and the world. In W. B, Walsh (Ed.), *Biennial review of counseling psychology* (Vol. 1, pp. 231–258). New York: Routledge/Taylor & Francis Group.

Institute of International Education. (2009). Record numbers of international students in U.S. higher education. Retrieved on July 11, 2011, from http://www.iie.org/en/Who-We-Are/News-and-Events/Press-Center/Press-Releases/2009/2009/-11-16-Open – Doors-2009-Internations-Students-in-the-US.aspx

Institute of International Education. (2009). *Open doors 2009: International students in the United States.* Retrieved from http://opendoors.iienetwork.org/?p=150649

Killian, K. D. (2001). Differences making a difference: Cross-cultural interactions in supervisor relationships. *Journal of Feminist Family Therapy, 12*, 61–103.

Leung, S.-M. A., Clawson, T., Norsworthy, K. L., Tena, A., Szilagyi, A., & Rogers, J. (2009). Internationalization of the counseling profession. In L. H. Gerstein, P. P. Heppner, S. Ægisdóttir, S.-M. A. Leung, & K. L. Norsworthy (Eds.), *International handbook of cross-cultural counseling: Cultural assumptions and practices worldwide* (pp. 111–123). Thousand Oaks, CA: Sage Publications.

Mittal, M., & Wieling, E. (2006). Training experiences of international doctoral students in marriage and family therapy. *Journal of Marital and Family Therapy, 32*, 369–383.

Mori, S. (2000). Addressing the mental health concerns of international students. *Journal of Counseling & Development, 78,* 137–143.

Mori, Y., Inman, A. G., & Caskie, G. I. L. (2009). Supervising international students: Relationship between acculturation, supervisor multicultural competence, cultural discussion, and supervision satisfaction. *Training and Education in Professional Psychology, 3,* 10–18. doi: 10.1037/a0013072.

Morris, J., & Lee, Y.-T. (2004). Issues of language and culture in family therapy training. *Contemporary Family Therapy, 26,* 307–318.

Ng, K.-M. (2006a). Counselor educators' perceptions of and experiences with international students. *International Journal for the Advancement of Counselling, 28,* 1–19. doi: 10.1007/s10447-005-8492-1.

Ng, K.-M. (2006b). International students in CACREP-accredited counseling programs. *Journal of Professional Counseling: Practice, Theory, and Research, 34,* 20–32.

Ng, K.-M., & Smith, S. D. (2009). Perceptions and experiences of international trainees in counseling and related programs. *International Journal for the Advancement of Counselling, 31,* 57–70. doi: 10.1007/s10447-008-9068-7.

Nilsson, J. E. (2007). International students in supervision. *The Clinical Supervisor, 26,* 35–47. doi: 10.1300/J001v26n01_04.

Nilsson, J. E., & Anderson, M. Z. (2004). Supervising international students: The role of acculturation, role ambiguity, and multicultural discussions. *Professional Psychology: Research and Practice, 35,* 306–312.

Nilsson, J. E., & Dodds, A. K. (2006). A pilot phase in the development of the international student supervision scale. *Journal of Multicultural Counseling and Development, 34,* 50–62.

Paige, R. M. (1990). International students: Cross-cultural psychological perspectives. In R. W. Brislin (Ed.), *Applied cross-cultural psychology* (pp. 161–185). Newbury Park, CA: Sage.

Pattison, S. (2003). Cultural diversity: Mapping the experiences of students on an international counselor training programme. *Counselling and Psychotherapy Research, 3,* 107–113.

Pedersen, P. B. (1991). Counseling international students. *The Counseling Psychologist, 19*(1), 10–58. doi: 10.1177/0011000091191002.

Peterson, D. M., Briggs, P. Dreasher, L. Horner, D. D., & Nelson, T. (1999). Contributions of international students and programs to campus diversity. *New Direction for Student Services, 86,* 67–77.

Singaravelu, H. D., & Pope, M. (Eds.). (2006). A handbook for counseling international students in the United States. Alexandria, VA: American Counseling Association.

Smith, S. D., & Ng, K.-M. (2009). International counseling trainees' experiences and perceptions of their multicultural counseling training in the United States: A mixed method inquiry. *International Journal for the Advancement of Counselling, 31,* 271–285. doi:10.1007/s10447-009-9083.

Takahashi, Y. (1989). Suicidal Asian patients: Recommendations for treatment. *Suicide and Life-Threatening Behavior, 19*(3), 305–313.

Wedding, D., McCartney, J. L., & Currey, D. E. (2009). Lessons relevant to psychologists who serve as mentors for international students. *Professional Psychology: Research and Practice, 40*(2), 189–193. doi: 10.1037/a0012249.

Yoon, E., & Portman, T. A. A. (2004). Critical issues of literature on counseling international students. *Journal of Multicultural Counseling and Development, 32,* 33–44.

Chapter 13

Programs of Counselor Training Outside the United States

For the first time in the series of editions that have made up *Counselor Preparation,* the 12th edition included a chapter about counselor training outside the United States and listed individual university data from foreign counselor education programs along with the individual university data from the United States. This first attempt encompassed countries from all over the world. The decision to expand *Counselor Preparation* to address training outside the U.S. was influenced by NBCC's increasing collaboration with counseling leadership in other countries, including leaders of training programs. It also was decided that future editions of *Counselor Preparation* would include international components. In this present edition of the book, the authors have decided to concentrate on trends in the counseling profession in Central and South America. This edition also presents data from other regions around the world. Future editions will highlight other world regions in the international chapter. The authors hope that continued international development will help define the future of the counseling profession.

COUNSELOR TRAINING IN CENTRAL AND SOUTH AMERICA
Sandra I. Lopez-Baez

Note: Information for this section was summarized from data provided by the following individuals: Dr. Cesar Vazquez (Puerto Rico), Lic. Omar García Miranda (Cuba), Dr. Antonio Tena Suck (México), Lic. María del Pilar Gracioso (Guatemala), and Lic. Andrés Sánchez Bodas (Argentina).

Twenty-six countries make up Central and South America. These include a number of autonomous republics, protectorates, and European territories. Although many of these countries share Spanish as a common language, their educational and cultural norms vary greatly. The development of the counseling profession is at various stages in these nations depending upon sociocultural needs, proximity to the United States and the influence of the North American educational system.

To gather data for this chapter, the author contacted ten individuals perceived to be leaders, trainers, and/or educators in the counseling profession in one or more Central and South American countries. Initial contact was made at conferences and via email, followed by an email asking the potential participants to participate by answering the questions sent to them. Participants were sent a total of four questions. The questions were

1. As best as you can, please describe the state of counselor training in your country (number of academic programs, types of specialty areas, etc.);
2. Briefly discuss some of the current issues related to credentialing of professional counselors;
3. What are some issues related to counselor licensure?
4. What regional trends and needs are there in your region as they pertain to counselor preparation?

Table 13.1 represents the information that was sent back to the author. It illustrates the diversity that exists in counselor training, ranging from bachelor's- to master's-level degrees. It also illustrates the developmental spectrum ranging from programs in the conceptual stages to those with clearly articulated curricula.

As Table 13.1 illustrates, there are academic programs offered through public as well as private universities and training institutes not affiliated with colleges or universities.

The information presented reflects the different stages of counselor training evolution in 5 of the 26 countries in Central and South America. The cultural reality of each country as it addresses the needs of its population is mirrored in the different training models employed as well as in the specialties that are currently offered and may be offered as different organizations develop and formalize counselor training.

TABLE 13.1 Counselor Training in Central and South American Countries

Country	Contact	State of Training	Number of Academic Programs	Specialty Areas	Credentialing, Including Licensure Issues	Counselor Preparation Needs
Puerto Rico	Dr. Cesar Vazquez	Train counselors since the 1950s at least partly due to U.S. proximity.	Nine universities offer master's degrees; two universities offer doctoral degrees (University of Puerto Rico and Interamerican University).		Until 2002 the Public Education Department certified professionals to practice in schools and private settings. In 2002, a licensure law was passed and implemented. The law regulates all counseling practice.	Professional training evolved from a post-baccalaureate professional diploma to a master's degree in Counseling.
Cuba	Lic. Omar García Miranda	In conceptual stage.	None. Plans are underway.	Since the 1940s guidance/vocational school professionals used the "test and tell" method for guidance activities with students.		Ideas for a curriculum that meets the needs of the local population are under development.

Continued

TABLE 13.1 (continued) Counselor Training in Central and South American Countries

Country	Contact	State of Training	Number of Academic Programs	Specialty Areas	Credentialing, Including Licensure Issues	Counselor Preparation Needs
Mexico	Dr. Antonio Tena Suck	At least one master's level academic training program.	One master's—a collaborative effort between the United States and Mexico through the University of Scranton and Universidad Iberoamericana.	Mental Health Counseling.		The role of counselors is not mentioned in the national mental health policy.
Guatemala	Lic. María del Pilar Gracioso	One known program.	Master's degree offered by the Universidad del Valle de Guatemala.	Psychological and Mental Health Counselor.	The bachelor's degree or "licenciatura" allows individuals to practice in their field.	
Argentina	Lic. Andrés Sánchez Bodas	There are academic programs offered through universities and training institutes.	Holos San Isidro: Centro Argentino de Psicología Humanística y Counseling [Argentine Center for Humanistic Psychology and counseling].			

Chapter 14

Expectations

Respondents from several schools provided information in this survey about changes anticipated in their programs. These included adding or deleting courses, changing accreditation status and other program changes. The following provides summaries of these planned changes.

COURSES

A program's curriculum must evolve with the counseling field. The continually expanding base of knowledge and best practices requires schools to alter courses from time to time. Twenty-three programs completed this section of the Data Collection Form. Respondents more frequently listed courses their programs might add; only one indicated that any courses might be dropped. The most common courses to be added to the curriculum included ones about addictions, crisis/violence counseling, crisis intervention, career/life planning, and supervision. Table 14.1 lists these responses.

ACCREDITATION STATUS OF PROGRAMS

As noted in earlier chapters, counselor preparation programs may seek accreditation.

Among respondents to this survey, school and community counseling programs led the field in attaining CACREP accreditation. Mental Health Counseling was listed as most likely to be applied for. Table 14.2 contains information from respondents on other specialty areas that are accredited or that plan to seek or drop accreditation.

TABLE 14.1 Planned Course Changes

Course Additions	Add
Action Research in School Counseling	1
Addictions	3
Advanced Theoretical Interventions	1
Advocacy	1
Career/Life Planning	2
Computer and Related Technology	1
Consultation	1
Counseling Children and Adolescents	1
Crisis Intervention	2
Crisis Management	1
Crisis/Violence Counseling	3
Electives	1
Evidence-Based Interventions. Adults, Crisis Management and Treatment	1
Grief, Trauma, and Disaster Counseling	1
Human Sexuality	1
Internet Use	1
Legal/Ethical Issues	1
Marriage and Family Counseling	1
Multicultural Counseling	1
Professional Issues/Ethics	1
REBT and Brief Therapy	1
Rehabilitation	1
Research and Program Management in Counseling	1
Substance Abuse Counseling	1
Supervision	2
Teaming	1
Theory Component	1
Course Elimination	
Technology	1

PROGRAM CHANGES ANTICIPATED

Schools offering counselor preparation programs anticipated further changes. One hundred programs answered this portion of the Data Collection Form. The most frequently anticipated changes were an increase in recruiting of diverse students and faculty and in the number of online courses. A summary of those responses is included in Table 14.3.

TABLE 14.2 Reported Accreditation Status of Programs

Accreditation Body	Program	Now Have	Applying for	Plan to Drop
CACREP	Career Counseling	4	—	—
	Clinical Mental Health Counseling	—	—	—
	College Counseling	7	—	—
	Community Counseling	45	1	3
	Counselor Education and Supervision	18	—	—
	Gerontological Counseling	1	—	—
	Marital, Couple, and Family Counseling/ Therapy	7	—	—
	Marriage and Family Counseling	2	—	—
	Mental Health Counseling	15	7	--
	School Counseling	58	5	--
	Student Affairs	3	1	1
	Student Affairs—Counseling	6	1	—
	Student Affairs—Professional Practice	4	—	—
CORE	Rehabilitation Counseling	10	—	—
AAPC	Pastoral Counseling	—	—	—

TABLE 14.3 Program Changes Anticipated by Departments

Anticipated Program Changes	Number of Programs Responding
Diversity recruiting of students	18
Diversity recruiting of faculty	14
Number of online courses	11
Other	11
Add Clinical Mental Health counseling program	10
National accreditation	7
Number of distance education courses	7
Number of off-campus courses	6
Faculty full-time equivalency	5
Financial aid	5
Admission requirements	4
Course offerings	3
Clinical supervision	2
Number of degree majors	1
Faculty	1

TABLE 14.4 Availability of Counseling Related
Programs at Same Institution Where Counselor
Preparation Programs Offered

Counseling Related Programs	Number of Programs Responding
Clinical Social Workers	11
Communications	12
International Studies	4
Marriage and Family Therapists	7
Organizational Behaviorists	3
Psychiatric Nurses	8
Psychiatrists	4
Psychologists	44
School Psychologists	3
Other	17

OTHER MENTAL HEALTH PROGRAMS

Several counselor education respondents also noted related programs offered on their campus. Psychology was the program most often listed. Frequencies of related programs are reported in Table 14.4.

SUMMARY

The data in this edition of *Counselor Preparation* is a summary of programs that responded to the survey in 2010. We have reported the responses to the survey without interpretation or comparison because the differences in the data collected have made meaningful comparisons impossible across the years. Also, a limit of the data in *Counselor Preparation* is that it is based on self-report.

Nonetheless, the dynamic nature of the counseling profession is apparent from this and other editions of this book. Exemplifying this is the inclusion of international programs in this edition of *Counselor Preparation* for the second time. We hope this continues to expand our understanding of counselor preparation around the globe.

In summary, many schools offering counselor education preparation are strengthening and revising their programs to meet the changing needs of the practitioner. More are incorporating technology into delivery systems, and more are populated with faculty who hold well-respected credentials. Unquestionably, these changes are shaping strong counseling professionals who are equipped to meet the needs of their clients. These developments also provide the foundation for the field's continued expansion, both nationally and internationally.

Data on Each Department

KEYS FOR PART D: DATA ON EACH DEPARTMENT:

M – Master's degree (i.e., M.A., M.S., M.Ed.)
S – Specialist degree (i.e., Ed.S., C.A.G.S.)
D – Doctoral degree (i.e., Ph.D., Ed.D.)
NP – Not Provided
CPCE – Counselor Preparation Comprehensive Exam
Assoc. Professor – Associate Professor
Full Prof. – Full Professor
F – Female
M – Male
Grad – Graduated
GRE – Graduate Records Examinations
MAT – Miller Analogies Test
Work Exp – Work Experience
Sem – Semester
Qtr – Quarter
Pract – Practicum
Intern – Internship
Comp – Comprehensive

AAMFT – American Association for Marriage and Family Therapy
AAPC – American Association of Pastoral Counselor
ABMP – American Board of Medical Psychotherapists
ABPP – American Board of Professional Psychology
ACS – Approved Clinical Supervisor
ACSW – Academy of Certified Social Workers
ASCH – American Society of Clinical Hypnotherapy
ATR – Registered Art Therapist
BCC – Board Certified Chaplain
BCD – Board Certified Diplomat in Clinical Social work
CAC – Certified Alcoholism (Addictions) Counselor

CADC – Certified Alcohol and Dependency Counselor

CADAC – Certified Alcohol and Drug Abuse Counselor

CCAS – Certified Clinical Addictions Specialist

CCDC – Certified Clinical Dependence Counselor

CCM – Certified Case Manager

CCMHC – Certified Clinical Mental Health Counselor

CDMS – Certified Disability Management Specialist

CESC – Certified Elementary School Counselor

CGP – Certified Group Psychotherapist

CLPC – Clinical Licensed Professional Counselor

CMFT – Certified Marriage and Family Therapist

CORE – Council on Rehabilitation Education

CPC – Certified Professional Counselor

CRC – Certified Rehabilitation Counselor

CRC-MAC – Certified Rehabilitation Counselor/Master Addiction Counselor

CSC – Certified School Counselor

CSSC – Certified Secondary School Counselor

CSP – Certified School Psychologist

CSW – Clinical Social Worker

CVE – Certified Vocational Evaluator

DCSW – Doctorate of Clinical Social Work

HSPP – Health Service Provider in Psychology

LCDC – Licensed Clinical Dependence Counselor

LCP – Licensed Counseling Professional

LCPC – Licensed Clinical Professional Counselor

LCSW – Licensed Clinical Social Work

LMFC – Licensed Marriage and Family Counselor

LMFT – Licensed Marriage and Family Therapist

LMHC – Licensed Mental Health Counselor

LMHP – Licensed Mental Health Professional

LP – Licensed Psychologist

LPC – Licensed Professional Counselor

LPCC – Licensed Professional Clinical Counselor

LPE – Licensed Psychological Evaluator

LPP – Licensed Psychological Practitioner

LSAC – Licensed Substance Abuse Counselor

LSC – Licensed School Counselor

LSSP – Licensed Specialist in School Psychology

LSSW – Licensed School Social Worker

LSW – Licensed Social Worker

MAC – Master Additions Counselor

MCC – Master Certified Coach

MFCC – Marriage, Family, Child Counselor

MFT – Marriage and Family Therapist

MHSP – Mental Health Service Provider

NCC – National Certified Counselor

NCCC – National Certified Career Counselor

NCGC – National Certified Gerontological Counselor

NCSC – National Certified School Counselor

NCSP – National Certified School Psychologist

PCC – Professional Clinical Counselor

PPS – Pupil Personnel Services

PPSC – Pupil Personnel Services Credential

RCC – Registered Clinical Counselor

RN – Registered Nurse

RPCC – Registered Professional Career Counselor

RPT – Registered Play Therapist

RPT-S – Registered Play Therapist-Supervisor

AL: The University of Alabama

Box 870231
Tuscaloosa, AL 35487-0231
United States of America
http://education.ua.edu/departments/esprmc/counselor-education/

Dean

James E. McLean, Ph.D.
College of Education
Box 870231
Tuscaloosa, AL 35487-0231
United States of America

Administrator

Joy J. Burnham, Ph.D., Program Chair
Box 870231
Tuscaloosa, AL 35487-0231
United States of America
(205) 348-2302; fax: (205) 348-7584
jburnham@bamaed.ua.edu

CSI Chapter, Name   Y, Rho Chapter
Regionally Accredited Y
Financial Aid   Y

Satellite Campus: N
International Students: N
Number of International Students: NP

Program Uniqueness

The majority of course work is completed in a traditional on-campus format.

Faculty Research

Faculty research interests include counselor development, rehabilitation counseling, counselor supervision, ethical/legal aspects of counseling, play therapy, and marriage/family counseling.

50% faculty in professional counseling practice.

Program Accreditation

CACREP: Community Counseling; **CACREP:** Counselor Education and Supervision; **CACREP:** School Counseling; **CORE:** Rehabilitation Counseling

Degree Programs

Degree	Program	Contact
M	Community Counseling	S. Allen Wilcoxon, Ed.D.
M	Rehabilitation Counseling	Jamie F. Satcher, Ph.D.
M	School Counseling	Karla D. Carmichael, Ph.D.
S	Community Counseling	S. Allen Wilcoxon, Ed.D.
S	Rehabilitation Counseling	Jamie F. Satcher, Ph.D.
S	School Counseling	Karla D. Carmichael, Ph.D.
PhD	Counselor Education	J J. Burnham

Distance learning: Y; 25% courses on-line

Other Counseling Related Programs

Clinical Social Workers
Communications
Marriage and Family Therapists
Organizational Behaviorists
Psychology

Faculty and Student Ethnicity

Faculty	**Master's**	**Specialist**	**Doctoral**
African-American	African-American	African-American	Asian
Caucasian	Asian-American	Asian-American	Caucasian
Latino/Latina	Caucasian	Caucasian	Latino/Latina
Native American	Latino/Latina	Latino/Latina	Multiracial
	Multiracial	Multiracial	

Faculty

Name			Highest Degree	Rank	Time	Credentials State Lic.	NCC	Email
Becerra	Michael	M	PhD	Assistant Professor	<21		Y	mbecerra@bamaed.ua.edu
Burnham	Joy	J	PhD	Associate Professor	<21		Y	jburnham@bamaed.ua.edu
Carmichael	Karla	D	PhD	Full Professor	22-40	Y	Y	kcarmich@bamaed.ua.edu
Hooper	Lisa	M	PhD	Associate Professor	<21	Y	Y	lhooper@bamaea.ua.edu
Leggett	Mark	F	PhD	Clinical Faculty	<21	Y	Y	mleggett@bamaed.ua.edu
Satcher	Jamie	F	PhD	Full Professor	22-40		N	jsatcher@bamaed.ua.edu
Wilcoxon,	S. Allen		EdD	Full Professor	22-40	Y	Y	awilcoxo@bamaed.ua.edu

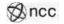

nbcc. Percent of faculty with NCC certification: 86%   ncc

Other Credentials Held By Faculty Members: AAMFT Approved Supervisor, AAMFT Clinical Member, Certified Elementary School Counselor, CRC, LMHC, LPC, RPT, RPTS

Enrollment and Admission Requirements

Degree	Program	Gender F	Gender M	Yearly Admit	Yearly Grad	GRE Total	MAT	Master	GPA	Work Exp	Letters	Interview
M	Community Counseling			14	9	1000	50	Y	3		3	N
M	Rehabilitation Counseling			14	10	1000	50	Y	3		3	N
M	School Counseling			11	7	1000	50		3		3	N
S	Community Counseling			19	9	1000	50	Y	3		3	
S	Rehabilitation Counseling			13	8	1000	50	Y	3		3	
S	School Counseling			11	5	1000	50		3		3	
PhD	Counselor Education			7	3	1000	50	Y	3	1	3	Y

Graduation Requirements

Degree	Program	Academic Hours Sem	Academic Hours Qtr	Clock Hours Pract	Clock Hours Intern	Thesis	Comp	CPCE	Oral	Portfolio
M	Community Counseling	60		100	600	N	Y	Y	N	Y
M	Rehabilitation Counseling	48		100	600	N	Y	Y		Y
M	School Counseling	48		100	600		Y			Y
S	Community Counseling	30			300	N	Y	N	N	Y
S	Rehabilitation Counseling	30			300	N	Y	N	N	Y
S	School Counseling	30			300	N	Y	N	N	Y
PhD	Counselor Education	72		300	600	Y	Y			

AL: University of North Alabama

UNA Box 5107
Florence, AL 35632-0001
United States of America
www.una.edu

Dean
Donna Jacobs
College of Education
UNA Box 5031
Florence, AL 35632-0001
United States of America

Administrator
Paul Baird, Professor and Chair
UNA Box 5107
Florence, AL 35632-0001
United States of America
(256) 765-4667; fax: (256) 765-5090
jpbaird@una.edu

CSI Chapter, Name   Y, Upsilon Nu Alpha Chapter
Regionally Accredited Y
Financial Aid   Y

Satellite Campus: N
International Students: N
Number of International Students: 0

Program Uniqueness

CACREP accredited under 2001 Standards. Strong emphasis on counseling skills development. Program provides practical support for students/graduates seeking to qualify for licensure and the national certification by administering the National Counselor Examination.

Faculty Research

Counselor supervision, the role of leisure activities in career development, academic success and failure among college students, advanced empathy skills, the instructional use of popular music and movies in counselor training.

Percent faculty in professional counseling practice: NP

Program Accreditation

CACREP: Community Counseling; **CACREP:** School Counseling

Degree Programs

Degree	Program	Contact
MA	Community Counseling	Paul Baird
MAEd	School Counseling	Paul Baird

Distance learning: Y; 15% courses on-line

Other Counseling Related Programs
NP

Faculty and Student Ethnicity

Faculty	Master's	Specialist	Doctoral
Caucasian	African-American		
	Asian-American		
	Caucasian		
	Multiracial		
	Native American		

Faculty

Name			Highest Degree	Rank	Time	Credentials State Lic.	NCC	Email
Baird	Paul		PhD	Professor	>81	Y	Y	jpbaird@una.edu
Loew	Sandra	A	PhD	Professor	>81	Y	Y	saloew@una.edu
Pearson	Quinn	M	PhD	Professor	>81	Y	N	qmpearson@una.edu
Townsend	Karen	M	PhD	Assistant Professor	>81	N	N	kmtownsend@una.edu

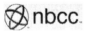 Percent of faculty with NCC certification: 50%

Other Credentials Held By Faculty Members: Certified School Counselor, LPC

Enrollment and Admission Requirements

Degree	Program	Gender F	M	Yearly Admit	Grad	GRE Total	MAT	Master	GPA	Work Exp	Letters	Interview
MA	Community Counseling	20	4	24	12	800	388	Y	3		3	Y
MAEd	School Counseling	5	1	6	3	800	388	Y	3		3	Y

Graduation Requirements

Degree	Program	Academic Hours Sem	Qtr	Clock Hours Pract	Intern	Thesis	Comp	CPCE	Oral	Portfolio
MA	Community Counseling	48		100	600	N	Y	Y	N	N
MAEd	School Counseling	48		100	600	N	Y	N	N	N

AL: University of South Alabama

UCOM 3800, College of Education
Mobile, AL 36688-0002
United States of America
www.southalabama.edu/coe/profstudies

Dean

Richard L. Hayes
UCOM 3614
Mobile, AL 36688-0002

Administrator

P. Irene McIntosh, Program Coordinator, Counseling Programs
UCOM 3800, College of Education
Mobile, AL 36688-0002
United States of America
(251) 380-2861; fax: (251) 380-2713
lmcintos@usouthal.edu

CSI Chapter, Name   Y, NP
Regionally Accredited   Y
Financial Aid   Y

Satellite Campus: N
International Students: Y
Number of International Students: 1

Program Uniqueness

All instructors have doctoral degrees and are active in community service. Several professors are involved in the state counseling association. Chair of the department is also chair of the Alabama Board of Examiners in Counseling. School counseling faculty is closely linked to the local school districts and in transforming school counseling. New graduate certificate program in mental health counseling just approved by university. Heavy integration of technology in teaching, advising and staying connected to alumni of the counseling programs.

Faculty Research

Research interests include at-risk youth, resiliency in youth, disaster counseling, ethics, supervision, and building community for youth and adults.

20% faculty in professional counseling practice.

Degree Programs

Degree	Program	Contact
M	Community Counseling	Irene McIntosh
M	School Counseling	Dr. Monica Motley

Distance learning: N; % courses on-line: NP

Other Counseling Related Programs

    Psychiatric Nurses
    Psychology
    Social Work

Faculty and Student Ethnicity

Faculty	Master's	Specialist	Doctoral
African-American	African-American		
Caucasian	Caucasian		
	Multiracial		

Faculty

Name			Highest Degree	Rank	Time	Credentials State Lic.	NCC	Email
Guest	Charles	L	PhD	Associate Professor	22-40	Y	Y	cguest@usouthal.edu
McIntosh	Irene		PhD	Associate Professor	>81		N	imcintos@usouthal.edu
McMahon	George		PhD	Assistant Professor	41-60		N	gmcmahon@usouthal.edu
Motley	Monica		PhD	Assistant Professor	>81		N	mmotley@usouthal.edu
Stefurak	James		PhD	Assistant Professor	41-60		N	jstufrak@jaguar1.usouthal.edu

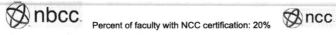 Percent of faculty with NCC certification: 20%

Other Credentials Held By Faculty Members: Certified School Counselor, Licensed Psychologist

Enrollment and Admission Requirements

Degree	Program	Gender		Yearly		GRE Total	MAT	Master	GPA	Work Exp	Letters	Interview
		F	M	Admit	Grad							
M	Community Counseling			14	10	0		Y	3	2	2	Y
M	School Counseling			12	9	0		Y	3		2	Y

Graduation Requirements

Degree	Program	Academic Hours		Clock Hours				Examinations			
		Sem	Qtr	Pract	Intern	Thesis	Comp	CPCE	Oral	Portfolio	
M	Community Counseling	54		100	600	N	Y				
M	School Counseling	48		100	600	N	Y				

AR: Arkansas State University

114 Cooley Drive
Jonesboro, AR
P.O. Box 1560
State University, AR 72467-1560
United States of America

Dean Don Maness, College of Education
United States of America

Administrator Loretta Neal McGregor, Chair
United States of America

CSI Chapter, Name Y, Beta Rho
Regionally Accredited Y
Financial Aid Y

Satellite Campus: N
International Students: Y
Number of International Students: NP

Program Uniqueness

Program tracks in college counseling, mental health counseling, rehabilitation counseling, school counseling and student affairs. Accommodating to part-time students through evening and summer classes.

Faculty Research
NP

% faculty in professional counseling practice: NP

Program Accreditation

 CACREP: School Counseling; **CORE**: Rehabilitation Counseling

Degree Programs

Degree	Program	Contact
M	Rehabilitation Counseling	Sharon Davis
M	School Counseling	Thomas Dodson
MS	Student Affairs and College Counseling	Nola Christenberry
EdS	Mental Health Counseling	Patrick Peck

Distance learning: NP; % courses on-line: NP

Other Counseling Related Programs

School Psychology

Faculty and Student Ethnicity
NP

Faculty

Name		Highest Degree	Rank	Time	Credentials		Email
					State Lic.	NCC	
Christenberry	Nola	PhD	Associate Professor	>81		N	nchriste@astate.edu
Claxton	Amy	PhD	Associate Professor	<21		N	aclaxton@astate.edu
Davis	Sharon	PhD	Assistant Professor	>81		N	sharondavis@astate.edu
Hall	John	PhD	Full Professor	22-40		N	jhall@astate.edu
Hestand	Philip	PhD	Director of Counseling and Training Center	<21		N	phestand@astate.edu
Howerton	Lynn	PhD	Full Professor	<21		N	howerton@astate.edu
Johnson	Robert	PhD	Full Professor	<21		N	rjohnson@astate.edu
Jones	Craig	EdD	Full Professor	22-40		N	cjones@astate.edu
Ochs	Lisa	PhD	Associate Professor	>81		N	lochs@astate.edu
Peck	Patrick	EdD	Associate Professor	>81		N	plpeck@astate.edu

Percent of faculty with NCC certification: 0%

Other Credentials Held By Faculty Members: NP

Enrollment and Admission Requirements

Degree	Program	Gender		Yearly		GRE Total	MAT	Master	GPA	Work Exp	Letters	Interview
		F	M	Admit	Grad							
M	Rehabilitation Counseling											
M	School Counseling											
MS	Student Affairs and College Counseling											
EdS	Mental Health Counseling											

Graduation Requirements

Degree	Program	Academic Hours	Clock Hours					Examinations		
		Sem Qtr	Pract	Intern	Thesis	Comp	CPCE	Oral	Portfolio
M	Rehabilitation Counseling	48	100	600		Y			
M	School Counseling	48	100	600		Y			
MS	Student Affairs and College Counseling	48	100	600		Y			
EdS	Mental Health Counseling	60	100	900		Y			

AR: Henderson State University

HSU Box 7774
1100 Henderson Street
Arkadelphia, AR 71999-0001
United States of America
http://www.hsu.edu/counselor-education/

Dean   Judy Harrison, Dean of Teachers College
HSU Box 7820
1100 Henderson Street
Arkadelphia, AR 71999-0001
United States of America

Administrator   R. Blari Olson, Chair
HSU Box 7774
1100 Henderson Street
Arkadelphia, AR 71999-0001
United States of America
(870) 230-5395; fax: (870) 230-5459
olsonb@hsu.edu

CSI Chapter, Name   N
Regionally Accredited Y
Financial Aid   N

Satellite Campus: N
International Students: N
Number of International Students: 0

Program Uniqueness

A program with six faculty. Ninety students in two programs. School and community counseling are CACREP accredited.

Faculty Research

Poetry therapy, parenting, cognitive behavioral counseling.

100% faculty in professional counseling practice.

Program Accreditation

CACREP: Community Counseling; **CACREP:** School Counseling

Degree Programs

Degree	Program	Contact
MS	Community Counseling	Other
MEd	School Counseling	

Distance learning: Y; 10% courses on-line

Other Counseling Related Programs

> MS in Clinical Mental Health Counseling
> MSE in School Counseling

Faculty and Student Ethnicity

Faculty	Master's	Specialist	Doctoral
Caucasian	African-American		
	Caucasian		
	Latino/Latina		

Faculty

Name			Highest Degree	Rank		Time	Credentials State Lic.	NCC	Email
Engllish	Linda		PhD	Associate	Professor	<21	Y	N	englil@hsu.edu
Kelly	Michael	D	EdD	Associate	Professor	<21	Y	N	kellym@hsu.edu
Moss	Rochell		PhD	Associate	Professor	<21	Y	N	mossr@hsu.edu
Olson	R.	B	EdD	Professor		22-40	Y	Y	olsonb@hsu.edu
Schmld	Richard	D.	EdD	Professor		22-40	Y	N	schmidr@hsu.edu
Weiner	Charles	A.	PhD	Professor		22-40	N	N	weinerc@hsu.edu

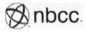 Percent of faculty with NCC certification: 17%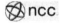

Other Credentials Held By Faculty Members: Approved Clinical Supervisor, Certified School Counselor, Licensed Psychologist, LMFT, LMFT Supervisor, LPC, LPC Supervisor

Enrollment and Admission Requirements

Degree	Program	Gender F M	Yearly Admit Grad	GRE Total	MAT	Master	GPA	Work Exp	Letters	Interview
MS	Community Counseling	45 5	30 25	790	380	Y	2.85		3	Y
MEd	School Counseling	10	10 10	790	280	Y	2.85		3	Y

Graduation Requirements

Degree	Program	Academic Hours Sem Qtr	Clock Hours Pract Intern	Thesis	Comp	Examinations CPCE	Oral	Portfolio
MS	Community Counseling	54	100 600	N	Y	N	N	Y
MEd	School Counseling	48	100 600	N	Y	N	N	Y

AR: Southern Arkansas University

100 E. University
Magnolia, AR 71754
United States of America

Dean   NP

Administrator   NP

CSI Chapter, Name   NP
Regionally Accredited NP
Financial Aid   NP

Satellite Campus: NP
International Students: NP
Number of International Students: NP

Program Uniqueness
NP

Faculty Research
NP

% faculty in professional counseling practice: NP

Degree Programs
NP

Distance learning: NP; % courses on-line: NP

Other Counseling Related Programs
NP

Faculty and Student Ethnicity
NP

Faculty
NP

Percent of faculty with NCC certification: NP

Other Credentials Held By Faculty Members: NP

Enrollment and Admission Requirements
NP

Graduation Requirements
NP

AR: University of Arkansas

136 Graduate Education Bldg
Fayetteville, AR 72701
United States of America

Dean   NP

Administrator   NP

CSI Chapter, Name   NP
Regionally Accredited   NP
Financial Aid   NP

Satellite Campus: NP
International Students: NP
Number of International Students: NP

Program Uniqueness
NP

Faculty Research
NP

% faculty in professional counseling practice: NP

Program Accreditation

CACREP: Community Counseling; **CACREP:** School Counseling;
CACREP: Counselor Education and Supervision

CACREP

Degree Programs
NP

Distance learning: NP; % courses on-line: NP

Other Counseling Related Programs
NP

Faculty and Student Ethnicity
NP

Faculty
NP

Percent of faculty with NCC certification: NP

Other Credentials Held By Faculty Members
NP

Enrollment and Admission Requirements
NP

Graduation Requirements
NP

AZ: University of Arizona

1430 E. Second St.
P.O. Box 210069
Tucson, AZ 87521-0069
United States of America
http://grad.arizona.edu/live/programs/description/146

Dean

Ron Marx, College of Education
1430 E. Second St.
P.O. Box 210069
Tucson, AZ 87521-0069
United States of America

Administrator

Sheri Bauman
Program Coordinator, School Counseling and Guidance
1430 E. Second St.
P.O. Box 210069
Tucson, AZ 87521-0069
United States of America
(520) 626-7308; fax: (520) 621-3821
sherib@u.arizona.edu

CSI Chapter, Name   N
Regionally Accredited Y
Financial Aid   Y

Satellite Campus: N
International Students: Y
Number of International Students: 1

Program Uniqueness

We use a variety of technology so that the program is accessible to non-traditional students. Our courses are specific to school counseling.

Faculty Research

Dr. Sheri Bauman studies bullying and victimization, cyber-bullying, and group work. Dr. Lia Falco studies gender and self-efficacy, and occupational decision-making in adolescence.

0% faculty in professional counseling practice.

Degree Programs
NP

Distance learning: Y; 75% courses on-line

Other Counseling Related Programs
NP

Faculty and Student Ethnicity

Faculty	Master's	Specialist	Doctoral
	African-American		
	Biracial		
	Caucasian		
	Latino/Latina		

Faculty

Name		Highest Degree	Rank	Time	Certifications		
					State Lic.	NCC	Email
Bauman	Sheri	PhD	Associate Professor	22-40		Y	
Falco	Lia	PhD	Assistant Professor			N	

nbcc.   Percent of faculty with NCC certification: 50%   ncc

Other Credentials Held By Faculty Members: Certified School Counselor, Certified School Psychologist, Licensed Psychologist

Enrollment and Admission Requirements
NP

Graduation Requirements
NP

AZ: University of Phoenix

	4605 East Elwood Street
	Phoenix, AZ 85040
	United States of America
	www.phoenix.edu
Dean	College of Social Science
	4605 E. Elwood St.
	Phoenix, AZ 85040
	United States of America
Administrator	Patricia L. Kerstner, Campus College Chair
	4635 East Elwood Street
	Mail Stop XCJA 201
	Phoenix, AZ 85040
	United States of America
	(480) 557-2179; fax: NP
	patricia.kerstner@phoenix.edu

CSI Chapter, Name   Y, Psi Omega Pi
Regionally Accredited   Y
Financial Aid   Y

Satellite Campus: NP
International Students: NP
Number of International Students: NP

Program Uniqueness

This is a program for working adults. Courses are at night and on weekends.

Faculty Research

Supervision, psychopharmacology, effects of hate crimes.

98% faculty in professional counseling practice.

Program Accreditation

CACREP: Clinical Mental Health Counseling; **CACREP:** Community Counseling

CACREP

Degree Programs

Degree	*Program*	*Contact*
MS	Community Counseling	Patricia L. Kerstner, Ph.D.

Distance learning: N; 0% courses on-line

Other Counseling Related Programs

> Bachelor of Science in Human Services
> Bachelor of Science in Psychology
> Master of Science in Psychology (online)

Faculty and Student Ethnicity

Faculty	**Master's**	**Specialist**	**Doctoral**
Asian	Asian-American		
Asian-American	Biracial		
Caucasian	Caucasian		
	Latino/Latina		
	Multiracial		
	Native American		

Faculty

Name			Highest Degree	Rank	Time	Credentials State Lic.	NCC	Email
Anderson	Shannon		PhD	Core faculty	61-80	Y	Y	1sassydoc@gmail.com
Babendir	Sheila		PhD	Core faculty	61-80	Y	N	
Carroll	Kim		PsyD	Adjunct	41-60	N	Y	
Doss	Sylvia		PsyD	Core faculty- lead faculty advisor	61-80	N	N	smdoss1211@aol.com
Downs	Mary		PhD	Adjunct	<21	N	N	ronmary@att.net
Floda	Tony		PhD	Core faculty	41-60	N	Y	tfloda@cox.net
Goulet	Wayne	L	EdD	Core faculty	61-80	N	Y	flyingwfg@cox.net
Kerstner	Patricia		PhD	Chair	41-60	N	Y	patricia.kerstner@phoenix.edu
Nixon	John		EdD	Director of Counseling and Training Center	41-60	Y	N	john.nixon@phoenix.edu
Snyder	Chad		PhD	Core Faculty	61-80	Y	Y	
Tanita	Glenn		PhD	Core Faculty	61-80	Y	Y	gtanita@aol.com
Weissman	Andrew		PsyD	Area Chair	61-80	N	Y	psydaz@hotmail.com

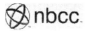

Percent of faculty with NCC certification: 67%

Other Credentials Held By Faculty Members: AAMFT Clinical Member, ACS, Licensed Psychologist, LPC, LPC Supervisor, MFT

Enrollment and Admission Requirements

Degree	Program	Gender F	M	Yearly Admit	Grad	GRE Total	MAT	Master	GPA	Work Exp	Letters	Interview
MS	Community Counseling	11	40	150	60	0		Y	2.5	2		Y

Graduation Requirements

Degree	Program	Academic Hours Sem	Qtr	Clock Hours Pract	Intern	Thesis	Comp	Examinations CPCE	Oral	Portfolio
MS	Community Counseling	60		100	600	N	N	Y	N	Y

AZ: University of Phoenix–Southern Arizona Campus

	300 South Craycroft Rd.
	Tucson, AZ 85711
	United States of America
	www.phoenix.edu
Dean	College of Social Sciences
	The University of Phoenix
	4605 E. Elwood St. MS AA-C704
	Tucson, AZ 85040
	United States of America
Administrator	Chad M. Mosher
	Campus College Chair for the College of Social Sciences
	Southern Arizona Campus
	300 South Craycroft Rd.
	Tucson, AZ 85711
	United States of America
	(520) 239-5208; fax: (520) 514-0948
	chad.mosher@phoenix.edu

CSI Chapter, Name   Y, Psi Omega Pi
Regionally Accredited Y
Financial Aid   Y

Satellite Campus: N
International Students: Y
Number of International Students: 3%

Program Uniqueness

The Master of Science in Counseling (MSC) degree program with a specialization in community counseling (CC) provides working-adult students the required knowledge and skills to become competent and ethical practitioners. The MSC/CC specialization provides a needed service to the community through collaboration with agencies and institutions and their personnel through the provision of continuing counselor education and programming. Students are involved in a variety of educational and clinical activities that prepare them to help their clients to achieve their potential. The program encompasses foundations of counseling and guidance including theories and their application with groups and individuals; assessment and evaluation; counseling and consultative relationships; and career planning for students and program development, implementation and evaluation. The program addresses critical issues facing counselors and offers supervised clinical experiences.

Faculty Research

Counselor identity; career issues; counselor education; supervision process; LGBTQ issues; multicultural issues in counselor training/competencies.

60% faculty in professional counseling practice.

Degree Programs

Degree	*Program*	*Contact*
MS	Community Counseling	Chad M. Mosher, Ph.D.

Distance learning: Y; 0% courses on-line

Other Counseling Related Programs

Criminal Justice (undergraduate)
General Psychology (undergraduate)
Human Services (undergraduate)

Faculty and Student Ethnicity

Faculty	**Master's**	**Specialist**	**Doctoral**
African-American	African-American		
Biracial	Asian		
Caucasian	Biracial		
	Caucasian		
	Latino/Latina		
	Multiracial		

Faculty

Name		Highest Degree	Rank	Time	Credentials State Lic.	NCC	Email
Dankowski	Ron	PhD	Core Faculty	22-40	N	Y	
Ellsworth	JoAnne	MEd	Adjunct	<21	Y	N	
Ferris	Dana	PhD	Core Faculty	<21	N	N	
Fortino	Juliet	MS	Adjunct	<21	Y	Y	
Goldman	George	PhD	Core Faculty	<21	N	Y	
Kurtz	Kelly	MS	Adjunct	<21	N	Y	
Lassiter	Rick	MS	Adjunct	<21	Y	N	
Levy	Lauren	MEd	Adjunct	<21	Y	N	
Matchett-Morris	Glenn	PhD	Core Faculty	22-40	N	N	
McKenna	Marta	MS		<21	Y	Y	
Mosher	Chad	PhD	Chair	<21		Y	
O`Connor	Sharon	MA	Adjunct	<21	Y	N	
Oppawsky	Jolene	PhD	Core Faculty	22-40	Y	N	
Quinley-Hayes	Deb	PhD	Core Faculty		Y	N	
Sadowsky	Joel	MA	Adjunct	<21	Y	Y	
Stromee	Vicky	MA	Core Faculty-Lead Faculty Advisor	22-40	Y	Y	
Wiggins	Fred	PhD	Clinical Faculty	22-40		Y	

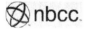

Percent of faculty with NCC certification: 53%   ncc

Other Certifications Held By Faculty Members: Approved Clinical Supervisor, Certified School Counselor, Licensed Psychologist, LMFT, LPC, RN, RPT, RPTS

Enrollment and Admission Requirements

Degree	Program	Gender F	Gender M	Yearly Admit	Yearly Grad	GRE Total	MAT	Master	GPA	Work Exp	Letters	Interview
MS	Community Counseling	75	25	100	60			Y	2.5	2		Y

Graduation Requirements

Degree	Program	Academic Hours Sem	Qtr	Clock Hours Pract	Intern	Thesis	Comp	CPCE	Oral	Portfolio
MS	Community Counseling	60		100	600	N	N	Y	N	Y

CA: California State University, Northridge

Department of Educational Psychology and Counseling
18111 Nordoff Street
Northridge, CA 91330-8265
United States of America
www.csun.edu/edpsy

Dean

Michael D. Eisner
College of Education
18111 Nordoff Street
Northridge, CA 91330-8265
United States of America

Administrator

Shari Tarver-Behring, Chair
Department of Educational Psychology and Counseling
18111 Nordoff Street
Northridge, CA 91330-8265
United States of America
(818) 677-2599; fax: (818) 677-2544
starver-behring@csun.edu

CSI Chapter, Name   N
Regionally Accredited   Y
Financial Aid   Y

Satellite Campus: N
International Students: Y
Number of International Students: 4

Program Uniqueness

Our graduate programs in counseling stress inclusiveness and collaboration in a supportive learning environment. Our courses are scheduled for two afternoon/evenings per week, which allows ample time for field experiences. Our faculty members have clinical and relevant counseling practice experience, with most continuing in that role, which provides a strong applied practice orientation to the graduate programs.

Faculty Research
NP

40% faculty in professional counseling practice.

Program Accreditation

CACREP: Career Counseling; **CACREP:** Marital, Couple and Family Counseling/Therapy; **CACREP:** School Counseling; **CACREP:** Student Affairs

Degree Programs

Degree	*Program*	*Contact*
MS	Career Counseling	Greg Jackson
MS	Marriage and Family Counseling	Stan Charnofsky
MS	School Counseling	Tovah Sands
MS	Student Affairs and College Counseling	Merril Simon

Distance learning: N; 0% courses on-line

Other Counseling Related Programs

Social Work
School Psychology

Faculty and Student Ethnicity

Faculty	Master's	Specialist	Doctoral
African-American	African-American		
Caucasian	Asian		
Latino/Latina	Asian-American		
Native American	Biracial		
Other	Caucasian		
	Latino/Latina		
	Native American		
	Other		
	Pacific Islander		

Faculty

Name			Highest Degree	Rank	Time	Credentials State Lic.	NCC	Email
Charnofsky	Stan		EdD	Professor	61-80	N	N	stan.charnofsky@csun.edu
Gehart	Diane		PhD	Professor		Y	N	diane.gehart@csun.edu
Gottfried	Adele		PhD	Professor	22-40	N	N	
Hanson	Charles		PhD	Professor	61-80	Y	N	charles.hanson@csun.edu
Laurent	Michael		PhD	Associate Professor	61-80	N	N	michael.laurent@csun.edu
Mitchell	Rie	R	PhD	Distinguished Professor		Y	Y	rie.mitchell@csun.edu
Rubalcava	Luis		PhD	Professor	61-80	N	N	luis.rubalcava@csun.edu
Sands	Tovah		PhD	Full Professor	61-80		Y	tovah.sands@csun.edu
Simon	Merril	A	PhD	Associate Professor	61-80	N	Y	merril.simon@csun.edu
Tarver-Behring	Shari		PhD	Professor		N	Y	shari.tarver.behring@csun.edu

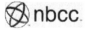 Percent of faculty with NCC certification: 40%

Other Credentials Held By Faculty Members: AAMFT Approved Supervisor, AAMFT Clinical Member, Approved Clinical Supervisor, Certified School Counselor, Certified School Psychologist, Licensed Psychologist, LMFC, LMFT, LMFT Supervisor, MFCC, MFT, PPS, RPCC, RPT, RPTS

Enrollment and Admission Requirements

Degree	Program	Gender		Yearly		GRE Total	MAT	Master	GPA	Work Exp	Letters	Interview
		F	M	Admit	Grad							
MS	Career Counseling	10	2	12	56	0		N	3	1	2	Y
MS	Marriage and Family Counseling	100	10	60	28			Y	3	0	3	Y
MS	School Counseling	20	10	30	12			Y	3	0	3	Y
MS	Student Affairs and College Counseling	18	6	12				Y	3	1	2	Y

Graduation Requirements

Degree	Program	Academic Hours		Clock Hours		Examinations				
		Sem	Qtr	Pract	Intern	Thesis	Comp	CPCE	Oral	Portfolio
MS	Career Counseling	60		100	600	Y	Y	N	N	N
MS	Marriage and Family Counseling	60		100	600	Y	Y	N	N	N
MS	School Counseling	55		100	600	Y	Y	N	N	N
MS	Student Affairs and College Counseling	60		100	600	Y	Y	N	N	N

CA: San Francisco State University

1600 Holloway Ave., Burk Hall 524
San Francisco, CA 94132
United States of America
www.counseling.sfsu.edu

Dean

Dean
1600 Holloway Ave., HSS Bldg, Room 204
San Francisco State University
College of Health and Human Services
San Francisco, CA 94132
United States of America

Administrator

Robert A. Williams, Chair
1600 Holloway Ave., Burk Hall 524
San Francisco State University
San Francisco, CA 94132
United States of America
(415) 338-2005; fax: (415) 338-0594
counsel@sfsu.edu

CSI Chapter, Name Y, Theta Chi
Regionally Accredited Y
Financial Aid Y

Satellite Campus: N
International Students: Y
Number of International Students: 2

Program Uniqueness

We prepare culturally competent, psychologically minded and emotionally grounded counselors in three degree programs: Master of Science in Counseling; Master of Science in Rehabilitation Counseling; and Master of Science in Marriage, Family, and Child Counseling (aka MFT). Within the M.S. in counseling, we offer career, college, gerontological and school specializations. Our department's faculty and the curriculum have been designed to aspire to achieve excellence in three core areas: multicultural competence, community partnerships and action research. Our faculty is locally, nationally and internationally recognized in their scholarly contributions to multicultural competence in counseling, social justice and health equity. Our faculty work provides a solid learning environment for students with disabilities, students from diverse ethnic and sexual orientations, as well as students from a range of socioeconomic groups.

Faculty Research
NP

% faculty in professional counseling practice: NP

Program Accreditation

CACREP: Career Counseling; **CACREP:** College Counseling; **CACREP:** Gerontological Counseling; **CACREP:** Marital, Couple and Family Counseling/Therapy; **CACREP:** School Counseling

Degree Programs

Degree	*Program*	*Contact*
	Professional Counseling	

Distance learning: N; 5% courses on-line

Other Counseling Related Programs
NP

Faculty and Student Ethnicity
NP

Faculty

Name		Highest Degree	Rank	Time	Credentials State Lic.	NCC	Email
Alvarez	Alvin	PhD	Professor	61-80	N	N	aalvarez@sfsu.edu

Percent of faculty with NCC certification: 0%

Other Credentials Held By Faculty Members: NP

Enrollment and Admission Requirements

Degree	*Program*	*Gender* F M	*Yearly* Admit Grad	GRE Total	MAT	Master	GPA	Work Exp	Letters	Interview
	Professional Counseling	40 10	50 50			Y	3		2	N

Graduation Requirements

Degree	*Program*	*Academic Hours* Sem Qtr	*Clock Hours* Pract	Intern	Thesis	Comp	*Examinations* CPCE	Oral	Portfolio
	Professional Counseling	60	280	660	N	N	N	N	N

CA: University of San Diego

5998 Alcala Park Counseling Program
School of Leadership and Education Sciences
San Diego, CA 92110
United States of America
http://www.sandiego.edu/soles/programs/counseling/

Dean

Paula Cordeiro
School of Leadership and Education Sciences
University of San Diego
5998 Alcala Park
San Diego, CA 92110
United States of America

Administrator

Lonnie Rowell, Director
University of San Diego
School of Leadership and Education Sciences
5998 Alcala Park
San Diego, CA 92110
United States of America
telephone: (619) 260-4212; fax: (619) 260-6826
lrowell@sandiego.edu

CSI Chapter, Name   Y, Sigma Delta
Regionally Accredited Y
Financial Aid   Y

Satellite Campus: N
International Students: Y
Number of International Students: 5

Program Uniqueness

The University of San Diego Counseling Program offers two program specializations. The 48-unit M.A. in Counseling with specialization in school counseling is CACREP accredited and also meets the requirements for the California Pupil Personnel Services credential in School Counseling. The 60-unit M.A. in Counseling with specialization in Clinical Mental Health Counseling graduated its first cohort in May 2010 and meets the requirements for the new California Licensed Professional Clinical Counselor (LPCC). Our program is focused on preparing counselors with the knowledge and skills to be effective in their specialization fields and to also be engaged in advocacy for their clients and for the profession. We have a culturally diverse student population. A unique feature is that all graduate programs in the School of Leadership and Education Sciences meet an internationalization requirement, and our program has offered graduate courses including a short study abroad experience for more than 15 years. Students in our program are able to get financial aid as well as access to other funding opportunities in our unit and on the campus. Our school counseling specialization has developed a model for collaborative action research that has been a core part of the program since 1999.

Faculty Research

The faculty members in the program are actively engaged in a variety of research areas. The counseling program has provided leadership in action research projects and hosts annually an

Action Research Conference. Faculty and students present at this conference as well as at other action research, counseling and educational conferences worldwide. Research areas addressed in the school counseling specialization include leadership and policy development in school counseling, school counseling outcome research and school reform. Faculty in the Clinical Mental Health Counseling Program focus research and presentations on forensic psychology, ethical and legal issues in professional practice, psychological assessment and provision of services for diverse client populations. Faculty and students have made presentations at conferences of ACA, ACES, AMHCA and the International Cross-Cultural Psychology Association. Program faculty has been active in getting counselor licensing legislation passed in California. Faculty also publish in the areas of internationalization of counseling programs and in effective practice with diverse client populations. Another faculty research area includes effective practices in higher education and college student development. School counseling faculty are published in the areas of action research, policy in school counseling and the application of Adlerian theory to school counseling.

28% faculty in professional counseling practice.

Program Accreditation

 CACREP: School Counseling

Degree Programs

Degree	Program	Contact
MA	Clinical Mental Health Counseling	Jonathan Raskin
MA	School Counseling	Lonnie Rowell

Distance learning: N; 25% courses on-line

Other Counseling Related Programs
NP

Faculty and Student Ethnicity

Faculty	Master's	Specialist	Doctoral
African-American	African-American		
Asian-American	Asian-American		
Caucasian	Caucasian		
Latino/Latina	Latino/Latina		
Pacific Islander	Pacific Islander		

Faculty

Name		Highest Degree	Rank	Time	Credentials State Lic.	NCC	Email
Gonzalez	Kenneth	PhD	Associate Professor	>81	N	N	kennethg@sandiego.edu
Johnson	Ronn	PhD	Associate Professor	>81	N	N	ronnjohn@cts.com
Martin	Ian	EdD	Assistant Professor		N	N	imartin@sandiego.edu
Nash	Erika	PhD	Assistant Professor		Y	Y	enash@sandiego.edu

Raskin	Jonathan	PhD	Full Professor		N	N	
Rowell	Lonnie	PhD	Associate Professor	61-80	N	N	lrowell@sandiego.edu
Zgliczynski	Susan	PhD	Associate Professor	>81	N	Y	zglnski@sandiego.edu

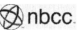 Percent of faculty with NCC certification: 29%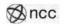

Other Credentials Held By Faculty Members: Approved Clinical Supervisor, Certified Elementary School Counselor, Certified School Counselor, Licensed Psychologist, LMHC

Enrollment and Admission Requirements

Degree	Program	Gender F	M	Yearly Admit	Grad	GRE Total	MAT	Master	GPA	Work Exp	Letters	Interview
MA	Clinical Mental Health Counseling	44	5	20	20	0		Y	2.75	1	3	Y
MA	School Counseling	44	8	22	22	0		Y	2.75		3	Y

Graduation Requirements

Degree	Program	Academic Hours Sem	Qtr	Clock Hours Pract	Intern	Thesis	Comp	Examinations CPCE	Oral	Portfolio
MA	Clinical Mental Health Counseling	60		100	600	N	Y			
MA	School Counseling	48		100	600	N	Y			

CO: Colorado State University

School of Education
Fort Collins, CO 80523-1588
United States of America
http://www.soe.cahs.colostate.edu/Graduate/MEd/CCD/Default.aspx

Dean
Carole Makela, Interim Director
School of Education
Fort Collins, CO 80523-1588
United States of America

Administrator
John M. Littrell, Program Chair
School of Education
Fort Collins, CO 80523-1588
United States of America
(970) 491-1061; fax: (970) 491-1317
John.Littrell@colostate.edu

CSI Chapter, Name   N
Regionally Accredited   Y
Financial Aid   Y

Satellite Campus: N
International Students: Y
Number of International Students: 1

Program Uniqueness

Indicative of the value placed on teaching in our master's program, three of the five full-time faculty members have received outstanding teaching awards in the past several years. Within the 2009-2010 academic year, the five faculty members published five counseling books.

Faculty Research   .

School counseling, school climate, GLBT issues, technology, brief counseling, metaphor, diffusion of innovation, ethical issues, group counseling, women's issues, spirituality and counseling, multicultural counseling.

20% faculty in professional counseling practice.

Program Accreditation

CACREP: Career Counseling; **CACREP:** Community Counseling; **CACREP:** School Counseling

Degree Programs

Degree	Program	Contact
M	Career Counseling	Rich W. Feller
M	Community Counseling	Sharon K. Anderson
M	School Counseling	Laurie A. Carlson

Distance learning: Y; 5% courses on-line

Other Counseling Related Programs

Counseling Psychology
Marriage and Family Therapy
Social Work

Faculty and Student Ethnicity

Faculty	Master's	Specialist	Doctoral
Caucasian	Asian		
	Caucasian		
	Latino/Latina		
	Pacific Islander		

Faculty

Name			Highest Degree	Rank	Time	Credentials State Lic.	NCC	Email
Anderson	Sharon	K	PhD	Associate Professor	41-60	N	N	Sharon.Anderson@colostate.edu
Carlson	Laurie	A	PhD	Associate Professor	41-60	N	N	Laurie.Carlson@colostate.edu
Feller	Rich	W	PhD	Full Professor	41-60	Y	N	Rich.Feller@colostate.edu
Kees	Nathalie	L	EdD	Associate Professor	41-60	Y	N	Nathalie.Kees@colostate.edu
Littrell	John	M	EdD	Full Professor	41-60	N	N	John.Littrell@colostate.edu

Percent of faculty with NCC certification: 0%

Other Credentials Held By Faculty Members: Licensed Psychologist

Enrollment and Admission Requirements

Degree	Program	Gender F	M	Yearly Admit	Grad	GRE Total	MAT	Master	GPA	Work Exp	Letters	Interview
M	Career Counseling	3	1	4	4	0		Y	3		3	Y
M	Community Counseling	2	1	3	3	0		Y	3		3	Y
M	School Counseling	12	1	13	13			Y	3		3	Y

Graduation Requirements

Degree	Program	Academic Hours Sem	Qtr	Clock Hours Pract	Intern	Thesis	Examinations Comp	CPCE	Oral	Portfolio
M	Career Counseling	52		100	600	N	Y	N	Y	N
M	Community Counseling	52		100	600	N	Y	N	Y	N
M	School Counseling	52		100	600	N	Y	N	Y	Y

CO: Denver Seminary

6399 S. Santa Fe Drive
Littleton, CO 80120
United States of America
www.denverseminary.edu

Dean
Provost Randy MacFarland
6399 S. Santa Fe Drive
Littleton, CO 80120
United States of America

Administrator
Fred Gingrich, Counseling Division Chair
6399 S. Santa Fe Drive
Littleton, CO 80120
United States of America
(303) 762-6954; fax: (303) 762-6976
fred.gingrich@denverseminary.edu

CSI Chapter, Name   NP
Regionally Accredited Y
Financial Aid   Y

Satellite Campus: N
International Students: Y
Number of International Students: 4

Program Uniqueness

The seminary context in which this program is located gives students an opportunity to integrate their professional counseling skills with spirituality. The Counseling Division operates a clinic on campus for community clients where students complete their practicum semester.

Faculty Research

Victim assistance; supervision; cross-cultural issues in supervision; brief therapy; attachment theory; MFT; complex trauma and abuse.

79% faculty in professional counseling practice.

Program Accreditation

CACREP: Community Counseling

Degree Programs

Degree	Program	Contact
MA	Community Counseling	Fred Gingrich
MA	Counseling Ministry	Janet McCormack
MDiv	Pastoral Counseling	Janet McCormack
MA	School Counseling	Debbie Edwards
DMin	Marriage and Family Counseling	

Distance learning: Y; 30% courses on-line

Other Counseling Related Programs
NP

Faculty and Student Ethnicity

Faculty	**Master's**	**Specialist**	**Doctoral**
African-American	African-American		
Caucasian	Asian-American		
	Caucasian		
	Latino/Latina		
	Multiracial		

Faculty

Name			Highest Degree	Rank	Time	State Lic.	NCC	Email
Beck	James	R	PhD	Senior Professor			N	
Cauthon	Roger		MDiv	Clinical Faculty			N	
Dempsey	Whitney		MDiv	Clinical Faculty			N	
Gingrich	Fred		DMin	Associate Professor and Chair			N	fred.gingrich@denverseminary.edu
Gingrich	Heather	D	PhD	Associate Professor	N		N	heather.gingrich@denverseminary.edu
Hasz	Monte		PsyD	Assistant Professor			N	monte.hasz@denverseminary.edu
Max	Dana		PhD	Clinical Faculty			N	
McCormack	Janet		DMin	Director of Chaplaincy and Pastoral Counseling	Y		N	jan.mccormack@denverseminary.edu
Moore	Reggie		MA	Instructor	Y		N	reggie.moore@denverseminary.edu
Nunnally	Clinton		MA	Clinical Faculty			N	
Showalter	Carrol		MA	Clinical Faculty			N	
Tiffany	Jeanne	B	M	Clinical Faculty			N	
Welch	Ron		PsyD	Associate Professor			N	ron.welch@denverseminary.edu
Well	Joan		PhD	Senior Professor			N	joan.wells@denverseminary.edu

Percent of faculty with NCC certification: 0%

Other Credentials Held By Faculty Members: AAMFT Approved Supervisor, Board Certified Chaplain, Licensed Psychologist, Licensed School Counselor

Enrollment and Admission Requirements

Degree	Program	Gender F	M	Yearly Admit	Grad	GRE Total	MAT	Master	GPA	Work Exp	Letters	Interview
MA	Community Counseling	17	40	70	50	0		Y	3		4	N
MA	Counseling Ministry	5	9	10	5	0		Y	2.5		4	N
MDiv	Pastoral Counseling	17	15	10	5	0		Y	2.5		4	N
MA	School Counseling	6	5	8	5	0		Y	3		4	N
DMin	Marriage and Family Counseling											

Graduation Requirements

Degree	Program	Academic Hours Sem	Qtr	Clock Hours Pract	Intern	Thesis	Comp	Examinations CPCE	Oral	Portfolio
MA	Community Counseling	66		125	600	N	Y	N	N	N
MA	Counseling Ministry	62		125	400	N	Y	N	N	N
MDiv	Pastoral Counseling	92			400	N	N	N	Y	N
MA	School Counseling	66			600	N	Y	N	N	N
DMin	Marriage and Family Counseling									

CO: The University of Colorado at Colorado Springs

Department of Counseling and Human Services
1420 Austin Bluffs Parkway
Colorado Springs, CO 80918
United States of America
www.uccs.edu/coe

Dean
LaVonne Neal
College of Education
University of Colorado at Colorado Springs
Colorado Springs, CO 80918
United States of America

Administrator
David Fenell, Professor and Chair
1420 Austin Bluffs Parkway
Colorado Springs, CO 80918
(719) 255-4096; fax: (719) 255-4110
david.fenell@uccs.edu

CSI Chapter, Name   Y, Chi Upsilon Sigma
Regionally Accredited Y
Financial Aid   Y

Satellite Campus: N
International students: N
Number of International students: 0

Program Uniqueness

The counselor preparation program delivered by the Department of Counseling and Human Services includes an emphasis on personal growth, self-awareness and adaptability as a person and professional. All students are enrolled in small lab groups facilitated by program graduates and supervised by core faculty in each of their first three semesters in the program. These small groups focus on skills development, self-awareness, personal and professional growth, and adaptability.

Faculty Research

Counseling military veterans and their families; girl bullying; effects of personal growth groups on counselor trainee development; play therapy effectiveness; school counseling innovation; multiculturalism; technology in counselor training.

50% faculty in professional counseling practice.

Program Accreditation

CACREP: Community Counseling; **CACREP:** School Counseling

Degree Programs

Degree	Program	Contact
M	Community Counseling	Dr. Joe Wehrman
M	Other-USAFA MA Program	Dr. David Fenell
M	School Counseling	Dr. Rhonda Williams

Distance learning: N; 0% courses on-line

Other Counseling Related Programs

Psychiatric Nurses
Psychology

Faculty and Student Ethnicity

Faculty	**Master's**	**Specialist**	**Doctoral**
Caucasian	African-American		
	Asian-American		
	Caucasian		
	Latino/Latina		
	Native American		
	Pacific Islander		

Faculty

Name			Highest Degree	Rank	Time	State Lic.	NCC	Email
Beecher	Catherine		MD	Instructor	61-80	Y	Y	cbeecher@uccs.edu
Fenell	David	L	PhD	Professor and Chair	22-40	N	Y	david.fenell@uccs.edu
Field	Julaine		PhD	Associate Professor	41-60	Y	Y	jfield@uccs.edu
McGuinness	Mari		MA	Instructor	61-80	N	N	mmcguinn@uccs.edu
Snyder	Beverly	A	EdD	Professor Emeritus	<21	Y	Y	
Wehrman	Joseph		PhD	Assistant Professor	41-60	Y	Y	jwehrman@uccs.edu
Weinhold	Barry	K	PhD	Professor Emeritus	<21	Y	N	
Williams	Rhonda		EdD	Associate Professor	41-60	Y	Y	rwilliam@uccs.edu

(above "State Lic." and "NCC" columns: **Credentials**)

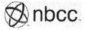 Percent of faculty with NCC certification: 75%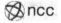

Other Credentials Held By Faculty Members: AAMFT Approved Supervisor, AAMFT Clinical Member, Licensed Psychologist, Licensed School Counselor, LPC Supervisor

Enrollment and Admission Requirements

Degree	Program	Gender F	Gender M	Yearly Admit	Yearly Grad	GRE Total	MAT	Master	GPA	Work Exp	Letters	Interview
M	Community Counseling	20	5	25	22				2.75	3	4	Y
M	Other-USAFA MA Program	4	16	20	20				2.75	10	4	Y
M	School Counseling	20	5	25	22				2.75	0	4	Y

Graduation Requirements

Degree	Program	Academic Hours Sem	Qtr	Clock Hours Pract	Clock Hours Intern	Thesis	Comp	Examinations CPCE	Oral	Portfolio
M	Community Counseling	60		100	600	N	Y	Y	N	N
M	Other-USAFA MA Program	45				N	Y	N	N	N
M	School Counseling	60		100	600	N	Y	Y	N	N

CO: University of Colorado, Denver

CB 106, P.O. Box 173364
Denver, CO 80217-3364
United States of America
http://www.ucdenver.edu

Dean   Lynn Rhodes

Administrator   Marsha Wiggins, Professor and Chair
CB 106, P.O. Box 173364
Denver, CO 80217-3364
United States of America
(303) 315-6332; fax: (303) 315-6349
marsha.wiggins@ucdenver.edu

CSI Chapter, Name   Y, NP
Regionally Accredited Y
Financial Aid   Y

Satellite Campus: Y
International Students: Y
Number of International Students: 5

Program Uniqueness

We have a strong focus on multiculturalism and diversity. We have a highly diverse faculty.

Faculty Research

Many faculty are involved in research regarding culture and diversity. One is interested in spirituality and counseling. Another focuses on career development.

10% faculty in professional counseling practice.

Program Accreditation

CACREP: Community Counseling; **CACREP**: Marital, Couple and Family Counseling/Therapy; **CACREP**: School Counseling

Degree Programs

Degree	Program	Contact
M	Community Counseling	Edward P. Cannon
M	Marriage and Family Counseling	Diane Estrada
M	School Counseling	Farah Ibrahim

Distance learning: N; 1% courses on-line

Other Counseling Related Programs

Communications

Faculty and Student Ethnicity

Faculty	Master's	Specialist	Doctoral
African-American	African-American		
Caucasian	Asian-American		
Latino/Latina	Caucasian		
Native American	Latino/Latina		
	Multiracial		
	Native American		

Faculty

Name			Highest Degree	Rank	Time	Credentials State Lic.	NCC	Email
Byers	Steven	R	PhD	Assistant Professor	>81		N	Steve_Byers@ceo.cudenver.edu
Estrada	Diane		PhD	Assistant Professor	>81		N	Diane_Estrada@ceo.cudenver.edu
Frame	Marsha Wiggins		PhD	Associate Professor	>81	Y	Y	mframe@ceo.cudenver.edu
Goalstone	Janet		PhD	Instructor	22-40	Y	N	Janet_Goalstone@ceo.cudenver.edu
Harding	Susan	S	PhD	Instructor	>81	Y	N	susan_harding@ceo.cudenver.edu
Helwig	Andrew	A	PhD	Full Professor	>81	Y	Y	Andrew_Helwig@ceo.cudenver.edu
Larsen	Patricia	A	PsyD	Instructor	>81		N	Pat_Larsen@ceo.cudenver.edu
Lasky	Joseph	F	EdD	Assistant Professor	41-60	Y	N	Joe_Lasky@ceo.cudenver.edu
Rutter	Philip	A	PhD	Assistant Professor	>81		N	Phil_Rutter@ceo.cudenver.edu
Williams	Carmen Braun		PhD	Associate Professor	>81		N	carmen_williams@ceo.cudenver.edu

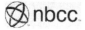 Percent of faculty with NCC certification: 20%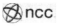

Other Credentials Held By Faculty Members: LMFT

Enrollment and Admission Requirements

Degree	Program	Gender F	Gender M	Yearly Admit	Yearly Grad	GRE Total	MAT	Master	GPA	Work Exp	Letters	Interview
M	Community Counseling	16	40	25	25	0	40	Y	2.75		4	Y
M	Marriage and Family Counseling			50	40	0	40		2.75		4	Y
M	School Counseling			45	40	900	40		2.75		3	Y

Graduation Requirements

Degree	Program	Academic Hours Sem	Academic Hours Qtr	Clock Hours Pract	Clock Hours Intern	Thesis	Examinations Comp	Examinations CPCE	Examinations Oral	Examinations Portfolio
M	Community Counseling	60		150	600		Y			
M	Marriage and Family Counseling	63		150	600					
M	School Counseling	63		150	600	N	Y	Y		

CO: University of Northern Colorado

McKee 248; Box 131
Greeley, CO 80639
United States of America
www.unco.edu/cebs/ppsy/

Dean   Eugene Sheehan
                     College of Education and Behavioral Sciences
                     McKee 125
                     University of Northern Colorado
                     Greeley, CO 80639
                     United States of America

Administrator   Heather Helm, Coordinator
                     McKee 248; Box 131
                     University of Northern Colorado
                     Greeley, CO 80639
                     United States of America
                     (970) 351-1630; fax: (970) 351-2625
                     heather.helm@unco.edu

CSI Chapter, Name   Y, Rho Epsilon
Regionally Accredited Y
Financial Aid   Y

Satellite Campus: Y
International Students: Y
Number of International Students: 8

Program Uniqueness

Our programs have a strong clinical focus and our graduates leave as well-trained clinicians. We have an on-site clinic equipped with audio-visual recording capabilities and one-way mirrors. The faculty and students form collegial professional relationships.

Faculty Research

White privilege; counselor education and supervision; women`s issues; adolescent issues; mentoring; play therapy; resilience; doctoral experience.

40% faculty in professional counseling practice.

Program Accreditation

CACREP: Community Counseling; **CACREP:** Counselor Education and Supervision; **CACREP:** Marital, Couple and Family Counseling/Therapy; **CACREP:** School Counseling

Degree Programs

Degree	Program	Contact
M	Clinical Counseling	Heather Helm
M	Couples and Family Counseling	Heather Helm
M	School Counseling	Heather Helm
PhD	Counselor Education	Linda Black

Distance learning: N; 0% courses on-line

Other Counseling Related Programs

Other
Psychology

Faculty and Student Ethnicity

<u>Faculty</u>	<u>Master's</u>	<u>Specialist</u>	<u>Doctoral</u>
Caucasian	African-American		African-American
Latino/Latina	Asian-American		Asian
	Caucasian		Caucasian
	Latino/Latina		Multiracial
	Multiracial		
	Native American		
	Pacific Islander		

Faculty

Name		Highest Degree	Rank	Time	Credentials State Lic.	NCC	Email
Athanasiou	Michelle	PhD	Full Professor	<21		N	michelle.athanasiou@unco.edu
Bardos	Achilles	PhD	Full Professor	<21		N	achilles.bardos@unco.edu
Black	Linda	EdD	Full Professor	>81	Y	N	linda.black@unco.edu
Cardona	Vilma (Betty)	PhD	Assistant Professor		N	Y	vilma.cardona@unco.edu
Clemens	Elysia	PhD	Assistant Professor		Y	N	elysia.clemens@unco.edu
Gonzalez	David	PhD	Full Professor	<21		N	david.gonzalez@unco.edu
Hannah	Fred	PhD	Full Professor	22-40	N	N	fred.hannah@unco.edu
Helm	Heather	PhD	Associate Professor	>81	Y	N	heather.helm@unco.edu
Hess	Robyn	PhD	Full Professor	>81		N	robyn.hess@unco.edu
Johnson	Brian	PhD	Full Professor	22-40		N	brian.johnson@unco.edu
Murdock	Jennifer	PhD	Assistant Professor	>81	Y	Y	jennifer.murdock@unco.edu
O'Halloran	Sean	PhD	Full Professor	22-40		N	sian.ohalloran@hotmail.com
Softas-Nall	Basilia	PhD	Full Professor	>81		Y	basilia.softas-nall@unco.edu
Wright	Stephen	PhD	Assistant Professor	>81	N	N	stephen.wright@unco.edu

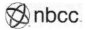 Percent of faculty with NCC certification: 21%

Other Credentials Held By Faculty Members: RPTS

Enrollment and Admission Requirements

Degree	Program	Gender F	Gender M	Yearly Admit	Yearly Grad	GRE Total	MAT	Master	GPA	Work Exp	Letters	Interview
M	Clinical Counseling	25	15	40	38	0		Y	3		3	Y
M	Couples and Family Counseling	9	6	15	15	0		Y	3		3	Y
M	School Counseling	9	7	15	15	0			3		3	Y
PhD	Counselor Education			6	6	1000		Y	3		3	Y

Graduation Requirements

Degree	Program	Academic Hours Sem	Qtr	Clock Hours Pract	Intern	Thesis	Comp	CPCE	Oral	Portfolio
M	Clinical Counseling	60		340	600	N	Y	Y	N	N
M	Couples and Family Counseling	66		150	600	N	Y	Y		
M	School Counseling	63		340	600					
PhD	Counselor Education	89		1270	1200	Y	Y		Y	

DE: University of Delaware

Human Development and Family Studies
Alison Hall West
Newark, DE 19716
United States of America
http://www.hdfs.udel.edu/content/counseling-higher-education-ma

Dean   Suzanne Austin
                        College of Education and Human Development
                        Newark, DE 19716
                        United States of America

Administrator   John. B. Bishop, Professor
                        Alison Hall West
                        Newark, DE 19716
                        United States of America
                        (302) 831-8544; fax: (302) 831-8776
                        Jbbishop@udel.edu

CSI Chapter, Name   N
Regionally Accredited Y
Financial Aid   Y

Satellite Campus: N
International Students: Y
Number of International Students: 1

Program Uniqueness

Either concentration usually requires two years of full-time study, excluding summer sessions. Strong emphasis on supervised practice. Several faculty members are also professionals in the Student Life Division.

Faculty Research

College student culture; student development; counseling in higher education; counseling center issues.

0% faculty in professional counseling practice.

Degree Programs

Degree	*Program*	*Contact*
MA	College Counseling	John Bishop
MA	Student Affairs Practice	John Bishop

Distance learning: N; 0% courses on-line

Other Counseling Related Programs

Psychiatric Nurses
Psychology

Faculty and Student Ethnicity

Faculty	Master's	Specialist	Doctoral
Asian	African-American		
Caucasian	Asian		
	Asian-American		
	Biracial		
	Caucasian		
	Latino/Latina		
	Pacific Islander		

Faculty

Name			Highest Degree	Rank	Time	Credentials State Lic.	NCC	Email
Beale	Charles	L	EdD	Assistant Professor	22-40	N	N	CBeale@udel.edu
Bishop	John	B	PhD	Full Professor and Director of the Master's Program	41-60	N	N	Jbbishop@udel.edu
Brooks	Timothy	F	EdD	Adjunct	<21	N	N	Tbrooks@udel.edu
Gilbert	Michael		EdD	Adjunct		N	N	mag@udel.edu
Kerr	Kathleen	G	EdD	Adjunct	<21		N	
Prime	Marilyn	S	EdD	Adjunct	<21	N	N	MPrime@udel.edu
Rarick	Susan	L	PhD	Assistant Professor	22-40		N	srarick@udel.edu
Sharf	Richard	S	PhD	Professor Emeritus	22-40	N	N	Richard.Sharf@udel.edu
Sharkey	Stuart	J	MEd	Professor Emeritus	<21	N	N	SSharkey@udel.edu
Tsukada	Karen	Y	PhD	Assistant Professor	22-40	N	N	

Percent of faculty with NCC certification: 0%

Other Credentials Held By Faculty Members: Licensed Psychologist

Enrollment and Admission Requirements

Degree	Program	Gender F	M	Yearly Admit	Grad	GRE Total	MAT	Master	GPA	Work Exp	Letters	Interview
MA	College Counseling	4	4	7	7	1050		Y	3		3	Y
MA	Student Affairs Practice	4	4	8	8	1050		Y	3		3	Y

Graduation Requirements

Degree	Program	Academic Hours Sem	Qtr	Clock Hours Pract	Intern	Thesis	Examinations Comp	CPCE	Oral	Portfolio
MA	College Counseling	48		140	300	N	Y	N	N	N
MA	Student Affairs Practice	48		140	300	N	Y	N	N	N

FL: Carlos Albizu University

2173 N.W. 99th Avenue
Miami, FL 33172-2209
United States of America
http://www.mia.albizu.edu

Dean   NP

Administrator   Diana Barroso, M.S., LMHC
                        Director of Master's Programs in Psychology
                        2173 N.W. 99th Avenue
                        Miami, FL, 33172-2209
                        United States of America
                        (305) 593-1223, ext. 143; fax: (305) 702-7806
                        dbarroso@albizu.edu

CSI Chapter, Name   NP
Regionally Accredited Y
Financial Aid   Y

Satellite Campus: Y
International Students: Y
Number of International Students: 30

Program Uniqueness

Carlos Albizu University is committed to training culturally sensitive professionals in the mental health field. The M.S. in Psychology program offers three majors: mental health counseling, marriage and family therapy and school counseling. Students may choose to pursue a dual major option.

Faculty Research

Cross-cultural and minority issues, psychotherapy outcomes, women's issues, history of ethnicity, anxiety sensitivity in the elderly, treatment of juvenile delinquents, systems family therapy, gay and lesbian issues, addictive behaviors, psychopathology, domestic violence, psychopharmacology, play therapy, bereavement issues, clinical work with children and families, alternative therapies, forensic issues.

95% faculty in professional counseling practice.

Degree Programs

Degree	Program	Contact
MS	Marriage and Family Counseling	Diana Barroso, M.S., LMHC
MS	Mental Health Counseling	Diana Barroso, M.S., LMHC
MS	School Counseling	Diana Barroso, M.S., LMHC

Distance learning: Y; 30% courses on-line

Other Counseling Related Programs

M.S. in Industrial and Organizational Psychology
Psy.D. in Clinical Psychology

Faculty and Student Ethnicity

Faculty	Master's	Specialist	Doctoral
African-American	African-American		
Asian	Asian-American		
Caucasian	Caucasian		
Latino/Latina	Latino/Latina		
Multiracial	Multiracial		

Faculty

Name		Highest Degree	Rank	Time	Credentials State Lic.	NCC	Email
Abraham	Kondoor	PsyD	Adjunct	22-40	Y	N	kvabraham@aol.com
Acosta	Odalys	MSW	Adjunct	22-40	N	N	oacosta@dadeschools.net
Barron	Irma	PhD	Associate Professor	>81	Y	Y	ibarron@albizu.edu
Barroso	Diana	MS	Full Professor and Director of the Master's Program	<21	Y	N	dbarroso@albizu.edu
Black	Ron	MS	Adjunct	22-40	N	N	ron@ce-classes.com
Campa	Fina	MS	Adjunct	<21	Y	N	fcampa@albizu.edu
Clark	Carol	PhD	Adjunct	22-40	Y	N	carollclark@bellsouth.net
Diaz	Tania	PsyD	Associate Professor	>81	Y	N	tdiaz@albizu.edu
DiDona	Toni	PhD	Associate Professor	>81		N	tdidona@albizu.edu
Finch	Teresa	PsyD	Adjunct	22-40	Y	N	
Garcia	Manolo	PsyD	Adjunct	22-40	Y	N	mgarcia1@mdo.edu
Haber	Karen B	PsyD	Adjunct	22-40	Y	N	
Hernandez-Hendrix	Nora	PhD	Adjunct	22-40	N	N	
Heyden	Edward	EdD	Associate Professor	>81		N	eheyden@albizu.edu
Jeanty	Guy	PhD	Adjunct	22-40	N	N	
Orta	Luis	PhD	Adjunct	22-40	Y	N	drorta@aol.com
Santana	Niurka	PhD	Adjunct	22-40	Y	N	drsantana@bellsouth.net
Stephenson	Edward	PhD	Adjunct	22-40	N	N	estephenson@fmuniv.edu
Valiente	Marilyn	PhD	Adjunct	22-40	Y	N	valientemp@aol.com

⊗ nbcc. Percent of faculty with NCC certification: 5% ⊗ ncc

Other Credentials Held By Faculty Members: Approved Clinical Supervisor, Board Certified Chaplain, CAC, Certified School Counselor, Certified School Psychologist, CSW, LCSW, Licensed Psychologist, LMFT, LMFT Supervisor, LMHC, LPC Supervisor

Enrollment and Admission Requirements

Degree	Program	Gender F	M	Yearly Admit	Grad	GRE Total	MAT	Master	GPA	Work Exp	Letters	Interview
MS	Marriage and Family Counseling	34	11	25	20			Y	3		3	Y
MS	Mental Health Counseling	12	40	50	20			Y	3		3	Y
MS	School Counseling	38	8	20	15			Y	3		3	Y

Graduation Requirements

Degree	Program	Academic Hours Sem	Qtr	Clock Hours Pract	Intern	Thesis	Comp	CPCE	Oral	Portfolio
MS	Marriage and Family Counseling	52		450		N	Y	N	N	N
MS	Mental Health Counseling	61		1000		N	Y	N	N	N
MS	School Counseling	49		240		N	Y	N	N	N

FL: Florida Gulf Coast University

10501 FGCU BLVD S.
Fort Myers, FL 33965
United States of America

Dean   Dean Marcia Greene
10501 FGCU BLVD S
Fort Myers, FL, 33965
United States of America

Administrator   NP

CSI Chapter, Name   NP
Regionally Accredited NP
Financial Aid   NP

Satellite Campus: NP
International Students: NP
Number of International Students: NP

Program Uniqueness
NP

Faculty Research
NP

% faculty in professional counseling practice: NP

Program Accreditation

CACREP: Mental Health Counseling; **CACREP:** School Counseling

CACREP

Degree Programs
NP

Distance learning: NP; % courses on-line: NP

Other Counseling Related Programs
NP

Faculty and Student Ethnicity
NP

Faculty
NP

Percent of faculty with NCC certification: NP

Other Credentials Held By Faculty Members
NP

Enrollment and Admission Requirements
NP

Graduation Requirements
NP

FL: Palm Beach Atlantic University

901 South Flagler Drive
West Palm Beach, FL 33401
United States of America
http://www.pba.edu/graduatestudies/counseling-psychology/index.cfm

Dean
Gene Sale
Dean of the School of Education and Behavioral Studies
901 South Flagler Drive
West Palm Beach, FL 33401
United States of America

Administrator
Lisa Stubbs
Director of the Graduate Counseling Psychology Program
901 South Flagler Drive
West Palm Beach, FL 33401
United States of America
(561) 803-2368; fax: NP

CSI Chapter, Name NP
Regionally Accredited NP
Financial Aid NP

Satellite Campus: NP
International Students: NP
Number of International Students: NP

Program Uniqueness
NP

Faculty Research
NP

% faculty in professional counseling practice: NP

Degree Programs

Degree	*Program*	*Contact*
MS	Clinical Mental Health Counseling	
	Marriage and Family Counseling	
	School Counseling	

Distance learning: N; % courses on-line: NP

Other Counseling Related Programs
NP

Faculty and Student Ethnicity
NP

Faculty

Name			Highest Degree	Rank	Time	Credentials State Lic.	NCC	Email
Dodson	Thomas		PhD	Full Professor	22-40	Y	Y	
Henry	Phillip		PhD	Full Professor	41-60	Y	N	
Rybalkina-Dietlin	Olga		PhD	Core Faculty	22-40		N	
Stubbs	Lisa		EdD	Chair	22-40	Y	N	
Vensel	Steven		MSW	Clinical Faculty	22-40	Y	N	
Virkler	Henry	A	PhD	Full Professor	61-80	Y	N	

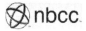 Percent of faculty with NCC certification: 17%   ncc

Other Credentials Held By Faculty Members: Approved Clinical Supervisor, LCSW, Licensed Psychologist, LMHC

Enrollment and Admission Requirements

Degree	Program	Gender F	M	Yearly Admit	Grad	GRE Total	MAT	Master	GPA	Work Exp	Letters	Interview
MS	Clinical Mental Health Counseling Marriage and Family Counseling School Counseling					0		Y	3		3	Y

Graduation Requirements

Degree	Program	Academic Hours Sem	Qtr	Clock Hours Pract	Intern	Thesis	Comp	Examinations CPCE	Oral	Portfolio
MS	Clinical Mental Health Counseling Marriage and Family Counseling School Counseling	60			1000	N	Y	Y	N	N

FL: Stetson University

421 N. Woodland Boulevard Unit 8389
DeLand, FL 32723
United States of America
www.stetson.edu/artsci/counselor

Dean
Grady Ballenger, Dean
College of Arts and Sciences
421 N. Woodland Boulevard
106 Elizabeth Hall
Unit 8396
DeLand, FL 32723
United States of America

Administrator
Brigid Noonan, Associate Professor and Chair
421 N. Woodland Boulevard
Unit 8389
DeLand, FL 32723
United States of America
(386) 822-8892; fax: (386) 740-3664
bnoonan@stetson.edu

CSI Chapter, Name   Y, Alpha Omicron Chapter
Regionally Accredited   Y
Financial Aid   Y

Satellite Campus: Y
International Students: Y
Number of International Students: 2

Program Uniqueness

Satellite campus in Celebration, FL, where most courses are held on the weekend to assist those working full-time. Students in DeLand are also able to take courses in Celebration and vice-versa.

Faculty Research
NP

100% faculty in professional counseling practice.

Program Accreditation

CACREP: Clinical Mental Health Counseling; **CACREP:** Marriage, Couple and Family Counseling; **CACREP:** School Counseling

CACREP

Degree Programs

Degree	Program	Contact
MS	Clinical Mental Health Counseling	Judith Burnett, Ph.D.
MS	Marriage, Couple and Family Counseling	Leila Roach, Ph.D.
MS	School Counseling	Page Thanasiu, Ph.D.

Distance learning: N; 10% courses on-line

Other Counseling Related Programs
NP

Faculty and Student Ethnicity
NP

Faculty

Name		Highest Degree	Rank	Time	Credentials State Lic.	NCC	Email
Burnett	Judith	PhD	Associate Professor	41-60	N	N	jburnett@stetson.edu
Noonan	Brigid	PhD	Associate Professor and Chair	41-60	Y	Y	bnoonan@stetson.edu
Roach	Leila	PhD	Assistant Professor	41-60	Y	Y	lroach@stetson.edu
Thanasiu	Page	PhD	Visiting Assistant Professor	22-40	Y	N	pthanasi@stetson.edu

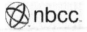 Percent of faculty with NCC certification: 50%

Other Credentials Held By Faculty Members: Approved Clinical Supervisor, Certified School Counselor, Licensed Psychologist, LMFT, LMHC

Enrollment and Admission Requirements

Degree	Program	Gender F	M	Yearly Admit	Grad	GRE Total	MAT	Master	GPA	Work Exp	Letters	Interview
MS	Clinical Mental Health Counseling					1000	410	Y	3		3	Y
MS	Marriage, Couple, and Family Counseling					1000	410	Y	3		3	Y
MS	School Counseling					1000	410	Y	3		3	Y

Graduation Requirements

Degree	Program	Academic Hours Sem	Qtr	Clock Hours Pract	Intern	Thesis	Comp	Examinations CPCE	Oral	Portfolio
MS	Clinical Mental Health Counseling	60		200	800	N	N	Y	Y	Y
MS	Marriage, Couple, and Family Counseling	60		100	600	N	N	Y	Y	Y
MS	School Counseling	57		100	600	N	N	Y	Y	Y

GA: Augusta State University

2500 Walton Way
Department of Educational Leadership, Counseling and Special Education
Augusta, GA 30904
United States of America
www.aug.edu/elcse/counseling

Dean

Gordon Eisenman, Dean of the College of Education
Department of Educational Leadership, Counseling and Special Education
2500 Walton Way
Augusta, GA 30904
United States of America

Administrator

Mary Jane Anderson-Wiley, Program Coordinator
Department of Educational Leadership, Counseling and Special Education
2500 Walton Way
Augusta, GA 30904
United States of America
(706) 667-4497; fax: (706) 667-4490
manders9@aug.edu

CSI Chapter, Name   Y, Gamma Rho Omega
Regionally Accredited Y
Financial Aid   Y

Satellite Campus: N
International Students: N
Number of International Students: 0

Program Uniqueness

As the second largest metropolitan area in Georgia, Augusta has a large urban population, but we also serve suburban and rural communities. From this unique vantage point, we recognize the critical need to address the economic, educational and social inequalities that exist in our community. As a result, we expect our students to develop a commitment of service to others, both for the prevention and remediation of life`s problems, and commit to the pursuit of excellence in the counseling profession.

Faculty Research
NP

0% faculty in professional counseling practice.

Program Accreditation

CACREP

CACREP: Community Counseling; **CACREP**: School Counseling

Degree Programs

Degree	Program	Contact
MEd	Community. Counseling	Dr. Richard Deaner
MEd	School Counseling	Dr. Paulette Schenck

Distance learning: N; 10% courses on-line

Other Counseling Related Programs

M.A. in Psychology

Faculty and Student Ethnicity

Faculty	Master's	Specialist	Doctoral
African-American	African-American		
Caucasian	Biracial		
	Caucasian		
	Latino/Latina		
	Multiracial		

Faculty

Name			Highest Degree	Rank	Time	Credentials State Lic.	NCC	Email
Anderson-Wiley	Mary Jane		PhD	Associate Professor and Director of Counselor Education	61-80	Y	Y	manders9@aug.edu
Deaner	Richard	G	PhD	Assistant Professor	>81	Y	Y	rdeaner@aug.edu
Schenck	Paulette	M	PhD	Assistant Professor	>81	N	N	pschenck@aug.edu

nbcc. Percent of faculty with NCC certification: 67% ncc.

Other Credentials Held By Faculty Members: Approved Clinical Supervisor, Certified School Counselor, LPC, LPC Supervisor

Enrollment and Admission Requirements

Degree	Program	Gender F	M	Yearly Admit	Grad	GRE Total	MAT	Master	GPA	Work Exp	Letters	Interview
MEd	Community Counseling	30	5	22	12	800	388	Y	2.5	1	3	Y
MEd	School Counseling	40	7	26	12	800	388	Y	2.5	1	3	Y

Graduation Requirements

Degree	Program	Academic Hours Sem	Qtr	Clock Hours Pract	Intern	Thesis	Comp	Examinations CPCE	Oral	Portfolio
MEd	Community Counseling	48		100	600	N	N	N	N	Y
MEd	School Counseling	48		100	600	N	N	N	N	Y

GA: Georgia Southern University

Box 8131 LTHD
Statesboro, GA 30460-8131
United States of America
http://coe.georgiasouthern.edu/lthd/counselored.html

Dean   Randall Carlson, Department Chair
                         Leadership, Technology and Human Development
                         Georgia Southern University
                         College of Education
                         Box 8131
                         Statesboro, GA 30460
                         United States of America

Administrator   Leon E. Spencer, Coordinator
                         Counselor Education Programs
                         Box 8131
                         Georgia Southern University
                         Statesboro, GA 30460
                         United States of America
                         (912) 478-5917; fax: (912) 478-7104
                         lespence@georgiasouthern.edu

CSI Chapter, Name   Y, Gamma Sigma
Regionally Accredited Y
Financial Aid   Y

Satellite Campus: N
International Students: N
Number of International Students: 0

Program Uniqueness

Program faculty is very diverse and has a strong research interest and focus on cross-cultural/multicultural counseling issues.

Faculty Research

Faculty is involved in cross-cultural/multicultural counseling issues. Faculty also hold leadership positions in state and national professional school and community organizations. The program faculty initiated the Southeastern Cross-Cultural Conference in Counseling and Education. This conference has consistently grown over the years with continued faculty support.

25% faculty in professional counseling practice.

Program Accreditation

CACREP: Community Counseling; **CACREP:** School Counseling;
CACREP: Student Affairs

Degree Programs

Degree	*Program*	*Contact*
MEd	Community Counseling	Leon E. Spencer
MEd	School Counseling	James Bergin
MEd	Student Services Higher Education - Counseling	Fayth Parks
EdS	Counselor Education Ed.S. in Counseling	James Klein Arline Edward-Joseph

Distance learning: Y; 7% courses on-line

Other Counseling Related Programs

Psychology

Faculty and Student Ethnicity

Faculty	Master's	Specialist	Doctoral
African-American	African-American	African-American	
Caucasian	Caucasian	Caucasian	

Faculty

Name		Highest Degree	Rank	Time	Credentials State Lic.	NCC	Email
Bailey	Carrie	PhD	Assistant Professor	22-40	Y	Y	cbailey@georgiasouthern.edu
Bergin	James	EdD	Full Professor	22-40	Y	Y	jim_bergin@georgiasouthern.edu
Edward- Joseph	Arline	PhD	Assistant Professor	22-40	N	N	aej@georgiasouthern.edu
Jackson	Mary	EdD	Professor Emeritus	<21	Y	Y	mjackson@georgiasouthern.edu
Parks	Fayth	PhD	Associate Professor	22-40	N	N	fparks@georgiasouthern.edu
Schulz	Lisa	PhD	Assistant Professor	22-40	Y	Y	lschulz@georgiasouthern.edu
Spencer	Leon E	EdD	Full Professor and Director of Graduate Program	<21	Y	Y	lespence@georgiasouthern.edu
Stewart	Patricia	PhD	Acting Assistant Professor	22-40	Y	N	pstewart@georgiasouthern.edu

 nbcc. Percent of faculty with NCC certification: 63% ncc.

Other Credentials Held By Faculty Members: Licensed Psychologist, Licensed School Counselor, LPC, LPC Supervisor, MAC, NCSC

Enrollment and Admission Requirements

Degree	Program	Gender F	M	Yearly Admit	Grad	GRE Total	MAT	Master	GPA	Work Exp	Letters	Interview
MEd	Community Counseling	26	3	15	15	0		Y	2.5		3	Y
MEd	School Counseling	39	2	20	10	0		Y	2.5		3	Y
MEd	Student Services Higher Education - Counseling	10	3	5	3	0		Y	2.5		3	Y
EdS	Counseling Education			15	5			Y	3.5			N
	Ed.S. in Counseling	18	4					Y				N

Graduation Requirements

Degree	Program	Academic Hours Sem	Qtr	Clock Hours Pract	Intern	Thesis	Comp	CPCE	Oral	Portfolio
MEd	Community Counseling	54		100	600	N	Y	Y	N	Y
MEd	School Counseling	48		100	300	N	Y	Y	N	Y
MEd	Student Services Higher Education - Counseling	48		100	600	N	N	N		Y
EdS	Counseling Education	30				N	Y	N	Y	N
	Ed.S. in Counseling	30					Y			

GA: University of West Georgia

Education Center Annex #237
Carrollton, GA 30118-4160
United States of America
http://coe.westga.edu/cep/

Dean

Kim Metcalf, Ph.D.
College of Education
UWG
Carrollton, GA 30118
United States of America

Administrator

Rebecca Stanard, Professor and Chair
Education Center Annex #237
UWG
Carrollton, GA, 30118-4160
United States of America
(678) 836-6554; fax: (678) 836-6099
rstanard@westga.edu

CSI Chapter, Name   Y, Gamma Zeta
Regionally Accredited   Y
Financial Aid   Y

Satellite Campus: NP
International students: Y
Number of International students: 3

Program Uniqueness

Department faculty are leaders in the national initiative to transform school counseling. Large and active chapter of Chi Sigma Iota (honorary society in counseling).

Faculty Research

Research interests of faculty are broad, culminating in many publications and presentations. Faculty is actively involved with significant agendas, leadership positions, service, innovative teaching and consultation.

0% faculty in professional counseling practice.

Program Accreditation

CACREP: Community Counseling; **CACREP**: School Counseling

Degree Programs

Degree	Program	Contact
MEd	Community Counseling	R. Stanard
MEd	School Counseling	R. Stanard
MEd	Student Affairs	R. Stanard
EdS	Professional Counseling and Supervision	R. Stanard
EdD	Professional Counseling and Supervision	Dr. Debra Cobia

Distance learning: N; 5% courses on-line

Other Counseling Related Programs

Psychology

Faculty and Student Ethnicity

Faculty	Master's	Specialist	Doctoral
African-American	African-American	African-American	
Asian	Asian-American	Asian-American	
Caucasian	Caucasian	Caucasian	
	Multiracial	Multiracial	

Faculty

Name			Highest Degree	Rank	Time	Credentials State Lic.	NCC	Email
Boes	Susan	R	PhD	Professor		Y	N	sboes@westga.edu
Cao	Li		PhD	Associate Professor	41-60	N	N	lcao@westga.edu
Charlesworth	John	R	PhD	Assistant Professor	>81		N	jcharles@westga.edu
Chibbaro	Julia	S	PhD	Associate Professor		Y	N	jchibbar@westga.edu
Cobia	Debra		EdD	Full Professor and Director of Graduate Program	61-80	Y	Y	dcobia@westga.edu
Hancock	Mary		PhD	Assistant Professor	41-60	N	N	mhancock@westga.edu
Painter	Linda	C	PhD	Associate Professor	>81	Y	N	lpainter@westga.edu
Parrish	Mark	S	PhD	Assistant Professor	>81	Y	N	mparrish@westga.edu
Slone	Mary	B	PhD	Associate Professor	41-60	N	N	mbslone@westga.edu
Snow	Brent	M	PhD	Professor and Associate VPAA	<21	Y	Y	bsnow@westga.edu
Stanard	Rebecca	A	PhD	Professor and Chair	22-40	Y	N	rstanard@westga.edu

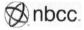 Percent of faculty with NCC certification: 18%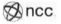

Other Credentials Held By Faculty Members: Certified Elementary School Counselor, Certified School Counselor, Licensed Psychologist

Enrollment and Admission Requirements

Degree	Program	Gender F	Gender M	Yearly Admit	Yearly Grad	GRE Total	MAT	Master	GPA	Work Exp	Letters	Interview
MEd	Community Counseling	10	5	15	15	900		Y	2.7		3	Y
MEd	School Counseling	45	5	50	50	900		Y	2.7		3	Y
MEd	Student Affairs	8	7	15	15	900		Y	2.7			Y
EdS	Professional Counseling and Supervision	10	5	15	15	900		Y	3		3	Y
EdD	Professional Counseling and Supervision	6		6	6	900		Y	3.5	3	3	Y

Graduation Requirements

Degree	Program	Academic Hours Sem	Academic Hours Qtr	Clock Hours Pract	Clock Hours Intern	Thesis	Examinations Comp	Examinations CPCE	Examinations Oral	Examinations Portfolio
MEd	Community Counseling	48		150	600	N	Y	Y	N	N
MEd	School Counseling	48			600	N	Y	Y	N	N
MEd	Student Affairs	42				N	N	N	N	Y
EdS	Professional Counseling and Supervision	27		100	150	N	N	N	Y	N
EdD	Professional Counseling and Supervision	111		300	300	Y	N	N	N	N

IA: The University of Iowa

338 Lindquist Center N.
Iowa City, IA 52242-1529
United States of America
http://education.uiowa.edu/crsd/

Dean   Sandra Bowman Damico
College of Education
459 Lindquit Center N
Iowa City, IA 52242-1529
United States of America

Administrator   Dennis R. Maki, Chairperson
338 Lindquist Center N.
Iowa City, IA 52242-1529
United States of America
(319) 335-5275; fax: (319) 335-5921
dennis-maki@uiowa.edu

CSI Chapter, Name   Y, Rho Epsilon
Regionally Accredited Y
Financial Aid   Y

Satellite Campus: N
International Students: Y
Number of International Students: 12

Program Uniqueness
NP

Faculty Research
NP

25% faculty in professional counseling practice.

Program Accreditation

CACREP: Community Counseling; **CACREP**: Counselor Education and
Supervision; **CACREP**: School Counseling; **CACREP**: Student Affairs;
CORE: Rehabilitation Counseling

Degree Programs

Degree	Program	Contact
M	Community Counseling	John Wadsworth
M	Rehabilitation and Mental Health Counseling	John Wadsworth

M	School Counseling	David Duys
PhD	Counselor Education	David Duys
PhD	Rehabilitation Counselor Education	Dennis Maki

Distance learning: N; 0% courses on-line

Other Counseling Related Programs

Clinical Social Workers
Communications
International Studies
Organizational Behaviorists
Psychiatric Nurses
Psychiatrists
Psychology

Faculty and Student Ethnicity

Faculty	**Master's**	**Specialist**	**Doctoral**
African-American	African-American		African-American
Caucasian	Caucasian		Caucasian
Latino/Latina	Latino/Latina		Latino/Latina
Native American	Multiracial		Multiracial

Faculty

Name		Highest Degree	Rank	Time	State Lic.	NCC	Email
Colangelo	Nicholas	PhD	Full Professor	<21		N	nick-colangelo@uiowa.edu
Duys	David	PhD	Assistant Professor	>81		N	david-duys@iowa.edu
Eichinger	Leanne	MA	Lecturer	<21		N	leanne.eichinger@doc.state.ia.us
Estrada-Hernandez	Noel	PhD	Assistant Professor	>81	N	N	noel-estradahernandez@@uiowa.edu
Harper	Dennis	PhD	Full Professor	<21		N	dennis-harper@uiowa.edu
Henfield	Malik	PhD	Assistant Professor	>81		N	malik-henfield@uiowa.edu
Maki	Dennis	PhD	Full Professor	>81	Y	Y	dennis-maki@uiowa.edu
O'Rourke	Barbara	PhD	Adjunct	<21		N	borouyke@blue.weeg.uiowa.edu
Portman	Tarrell	PhD	Associate Professor	>81		Y	tarrell-portman@uiowa.edu
Saunders	Jodi	PhD	Associate Professor	>81	N	N	jodi-saunders@uiowa.edu
Smith	Carol	PhD	Clinical Faculty	>81	Y	Y	carol-smith@uiowa.edu
Stachowiak	James	MS	Adjunct	<21		N	james-stachowiak@uiowa.edu
Tarvydas	Vilia	PhD	Full Professor		Y	N	vilia-tarvydas@uiowa.edu
Teahen	Peter	MA	Adjunct	<21		N	
Townsend	Orville	MA	Adjunct	<21		N	
Wadsworth	John	PhD	Associate Professor		Y	N	john-s-wadsworth@uiowa.edu
Wood	Susannah	PhD	Assistant Professor	>81		Y	susannah-wood@uiowa.edu
Zalenski	Anne	PhD	Adjunct	<21		N	anne-zalenski@uiowa.edu

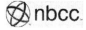   Percent of faculty with NCC certification: 22%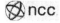

Other Credentials Held By Faculty Members: Approved Clinical Supervisor, Certified Elementary School Counselor, Certified School Counselor, Certified Secondary School Counselor, CRC, Licensed School Counselor, LMHC, LPC

Enrollment and Admission Requirements

Degree	Program	Gender		Yearly		GRE Total	MAT	Master	GPA	Work Exp	Letters	Interview
		F	M	Admit	Grad							
M	Community Counseling	28	2	15	15	0			3	1	3	Y
M	Rehabilitation and Mental Health Counseling	25	5	15	15	0			3	1	3	Y
M	School Counseling			15	15	0			3		3	Y
PhD	Counselor Education	8	7	3	3	1000		Y	3	1	3	Y
PhD	Rehabilitation Counselor Education	6	3	3	3	1000		Y	3		3	Y

Graduation Requirements

Degree	Program	Academic Hours		Clock Hours		Examinations				
		Sem	Qtr	Pract	Intern	Thesis	Comp	CPCE	Oral	Portfolio
M	Community Counseling	60		360	600	N	Y			
M	Rehabilitation and Mental Health Counseling	60		360	600		Y			
M	School Counseling	54		100	600	N	Y	N	N	N
PhD	Counselor Education	96		180	600	Y	Y		Y	
PhD	Rehabilitation Counselor Education	96		180		Y	Y		Y	

ID: Boise State University

1910 University Avenue
Education 611
Boise, ID 83725
United States of America
http://education.boisestate.edu/counseling

Dean
Diane Boothe
College of Education
1910 University Avenue
Boise, ID 83725
United States of America

Administrator
Bobbie Birdsall, Chair
1910 University Avenue
Education 611
Boise, ID 83725
United States of America
(208) 426-1219; fax: NP
bbirdsa@boisestate.edu

CSI Chapter, Name   Y, Beta Sigma Upsilon
Regionally Accredited Y
Financial Aid   Y

Satellite Campus: N
International Students: Y
Number of International Students: 1

Program Uniqueness

Sixty-credit degree focusing on school counseling with optional addiction studies track, leading to state certification and/or licensure and addictions credentials. Courses offered primarily nights and weekends to accommodate employed persons. Companion institution to The Education Trust counseling reform initiative.

Faculty Research

Bobbie Birdsall's (NCC, NCSC, LPCP) research areas are family counseling in school settings, spirituality in counseling and school counseling reform. She is an appointed member of the Idaho Licensure Board. Ken Coll's (NCC, LPCP) research areas are addictions prevention, effective assessment and interventions for adolescents, and outcome based evaluation. He is a successful grant writer in Addictions Studies. Maggie Miller's (NBSC, LPC, LCPC) research areas are equity and ethical practice in a multicultural society and the role of counselors in education reform. She is an appointed member of the Idaho Counseling Advisory Committee. AnneMarie Nelson's (LPC) research areas are story-telling and mythology as tools in counseling. She is current president of the Idaho Psychological Association.

100% faculty in professional counseling practice.

Program Accreditation

CACREP: School Counseling

Degree Programs

Degree	Program	Contact
M	Addictions Counseling School Counseling	Dr. Bobbie Birdsall

Distance learning: N; 0% courses on-line

Other Counseling Related Programs

Clinical Social Workers
Communications
Other

Faculty and Student Ethnicity

Faculty	Master's	Specialist	Doctoral
Caucasian	African-American		
	Asian-American		
	Caucasian		
	Latino/Latina		
	Native American		

Faculty

Name			Highest Degree	Rank	Time	Credentials State Lic.	NCC	Email
Birdsall	Bobbie		PhD	Associate Professor	>81	Y	Y	bbirdsa@boisestate.edu
Coll	Ken	M	PhD	Full Professor	41-60	Y	Y	kcoll@boisestate.edu
Miller	Maggie		PhD	Full Professor	>81	Y	N	mmiller@boisestate.edu
Nelson	AnneMarie		PhD	Associate Professor	>81	Y	N	anelson@boisestate.edu

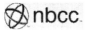   Percent of faculty with NCC certification: 50%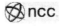

Other Credentials Held By Faculty Members
NP

Enrollment and Admission Requirements

Degree	Program	Gender F	Gender M	Yearly Admit	Yearly Grad	GRE Total	MAT	Master	GPA	Work Exp	Letters	Interview
M	Addictions Counseling	22	4	26	20	0		Y	3		3	Y
	School Counseling	22	4	26	22							

Graduation Requirements

Degree	Program	Academic Hours Sem	Qtr	Clock Hours Pract	Intern	Thesis	Comp	Examinations CPCE	Oral	Portfolio
M	Addictions Counseling	60		100	700	N	N	Y	N	Y
	School Counseling									

IL: Loyola University Chicago

820 North Michigan Avenue
Chicago, IL 60611
United States of America
luc.edu

Dean   David Prasse
820 North Michigan Avenue
11th Floor, Lewis Towers
Chicago, IL 60611
United States of America

Administrator   Anita Thomas, Graduate Program Director
Chicago, IL 60611
United States of America
(312) 915-6836; fax: (312) 915-6690
athoma9@luc.edu

CSI Chapter, Name   N
Regionally Accredited   Y
Financial Aid   Y

Satellite Campus: N
International Students: Y
Number of International Students: 2

Program Uniqueness
NP

Faculty Research
NP

% faculty in professional counseling practice: NP

Degree Programs

Degree	*Program*	*Contact*
MEd	Community Counseling	Dr. Anita Thomas
MA	Community Counseling	Dr. Anita Thomas
MEd	School Counseling	Dr. Anita Thomas
	Counseling Psychology	Dr. Anita Thomas

Distance learning: N; % courses on-line: NP

Other Counseling Related Programs
NP

Faculty and Student Ethnicity
NP

Faculty

Name			Highest Degree	Rank	Time	Credentials State Lic.	NCC	Email
Brown	Steven	D	PhD	Professor		N	N	sbrown@luc.edu
Mildner	Carolyn		PhD	Assistant Professor		N	N	cmildn@luc.edu
Thomas	Anita	J	PhD	Associate Professor		N	N	athoma9@luc.edu
Vera	Elizabeth		PhD	Professor		N	N	evera@luc.edu
Yoon	Eunju		PhD	Assistant Professor		N	N	eyoon@luc.edu

Percent of faculty with NCC certification: 0%

Other Credentials Held By Faculty Members: Licensed Psychologist

Enrollment and Admission Requirements

Degree	Program	Gender F	M	Yearly Admit	Grad	GRE Total	MAT	Master	GPA	Work Exp	Letters	Interview
MEd	Community Counseling	17	3	50	30	1100		Y	3	0	3	N
MA	Community Counseling	10	0	50	10	1100		Y	3			N
MEd	School Counseling	19	5	50	20							
	Counseling Psychology	18	6	4	6	1200		Y	3	2	3	Y

Graduation Requirements

Degree	Program	Academic Hours Sem	Qtr	Clock Hours Pract	Intern	Thesis	Comp	Examinations CPCE	Oral	Portfolio
MEd	Community Counseling	48		700		N	Y	Y	N	N
MA	Community Counseling	48		700		N	Y	Y	N	N
MEd	School Counseling									
	Counseling Psychology	66		1000	2000	Y	Y	N	Y	

IN: Ball State University

Teachers College 622
Muncie, IN 47306-0585
United States of America
www.bsu.edu/counselingpsych

Dean
Roy A. Weaver
Teachers College
Ball State University
Muncie, IN 47306
United States of America

Administrator
Sharon L. Bowman, Chairperson
Teachers College 622
Ball State University
Muncie IN, 47306-0585
United States of America
(765) 285-8040; fax: (765) 285-2067
sbowman@bsu.edu

CSI Chapter, Name   NP
Regionally Accredited Y
Financial Aid   Y

Satellite Campus: NP
International Students: NP
Number of International Students: NP

Program Uniqueness

Large faculty with diverse interests; balance of research and experiential components.

Faculty Research

Multicultural Issues; psycho-social oncology.

33% faculty in professional counseling practice.

Program Accreditation

CACREP: Community Counseling; **CACREP:** School Counseling; **CORE:** Rehabilitation Counseling

Degree Programs

Degree	Program	Contact
M	Community Counseling	Kristin M. Perrone-McGovern
M	Mental Health Counseling	Kristin M. Perrone-McGovern
M	Rehabilitation Counseling	Molly K. Tschopp

M	School Counseling	Charlene Alexander
PhD	Other	Lawrence Gerstein

Distance learning: No; % courses on-line: NP

Other Counseling Related Programs
NP

Faculty and Student Ethnicity
NP

Faculty

Name			Highest Degree	Rank	Time	Credentials State Lic.	NCC	Email
Aegisdottir	Stefania		PhD	Assistant Professor	61-80	N	N	stefaegis@bsu.edu
Alexander	Charlene	M	PhD	Associate Professor	61-80	N	N	calexander@bsu.edu
Bowman	Sharon	L	PhD	Full Professor	41-60	N	N	sbowman@bsu.edu
Dixon	David	N	PhD	Full Professor	61-80	N	N	ddixon@bsu.edu
Gerstein	Lawrence	H	PhD	Full Professor	61-80	N	N	rangzen@aol.com
Kruczek	Theresa	A	PhD	Associate Professor	61-80	N	N	tkruczek@bsu.edu
Nicholas	Donald	R	PhD	Full Professor	61-80	N	N	dnichola@bsu.edu
Perrone-McGovern	Kristin	M	PhD	Associate Professor	61-80	N	N	kperrone@bsu.edu
Spengler	Paul	M	PhD	Associate Professor	61-80	N	N	pspengle@bsu.edu
Tschopp	Molly	K	PhD	Assistant Professor	61-80	N	N	mktschopp@bsu.edu
White	Michael	J	PhD	Full Professor	61-80	N	N	00mjwhite@bsu.edu

Percent of faculty with NCC certification: 0%

Other Credentials Held By Faculty Members: Certified School Counselor, CRC, Licensed Psychologist, LMHC

Enrollment and Admission Requirements

Degree	Program	Gender F	M	Yearly Admit	Grad	GRE Total	MAT	Master	GPA	Work Exp	Letters	Interview
M	Community Counseling	7	3	10	10	900		Y	2.75		3	N
M	Mental Health Counseling	15	5	20	15	900		Y	2.75		3	N
M	Rehabilitation Counseling	5	3	8	7	900			2.75		3	N
M	School Counseling	10	2	12	10	900			2.75		3	N
PhD	Other	5	5	10	7	1000		N			3	Y

Graduation Requirements

Degree	Program	Academic Hours Sem	Qtr	Clock Hours Pract	Intern	Thesis	Comp	Examinations CPCE	Oral	Portfolio
M	Community Counseling	48		200	600	N	N	Y	N	N
M	Mental Health Counseling	60		200	900	N	N	Y	N	N
M	Rehabilitation Counseling	48		100	600	N	N	Y	N	N
M	School Counseling	48		200	600	N	N	N	N	Y
PhD	Other	97		400	1500	Y	Y	N	Y	Y

KS: Kansas State University

1100 Mid-Campus Dr., Rm. 369
Manhattan, KS 66506-5312
United States of America
http://coe.ksu.edu

Dean Michael C. Holen

Administrator Ken Hughey, Department Chair
1100 Mid-Campus Dr., Rm. 369
Manhattan, KS 66506-5312
United States of America
(785) 532-5541; fax: (785) 532-7304
khughey@ksu.edu

CSI Chapter, Name N
Regionally Accredited Y
Financial Aid Y

Satellite Campus: N
International Students: N
Number of International Students: 0

Program Uniqueness

Both the M.S. in School Counseling and the Ph.D. in Counselor Education and Supervision are
CACREP accredited.

Faculty Research

Career development, counseling support for culturally and linguistically diverse students,
counseling supervision, testing in counseling, multicultural counseling, sports and exercise
psychology, school counseling, career advising, spirituality and religion in higher education,
history and philosophy of higher education, wellness.

0% faculty in professional counseling practice.

Program Accreditation

CACREP: Counselor Education and Supervision; **CACREP:** School Counseling

Degree Programs

Degree	Program	Contact
MS	Academic Advising	Dr. Ken Hughey
Other	Academic Advising Certificate	Dr. Ken Hughey
MS	School Counseling	Dr. Judith Hughey
MS	Student Affairs	Dr. Christy Moran
MS	Student Services in Intercollegiate Athletics	Dr. Brandonn Harris
PhD	Counselor Education	Dr. Ken Hughey
PhD	Student Affairs	Dr. Doris Wright-Carroll

Distance learning: Y; 35% courses on-line

Other Counseling Related Programs

Marriage and Family Therapists

Faculty and Student Ethnicity

Faculty	**Master's**	**Specialist**	**Doctoral**
African-American	African-American		African-American
Caucasian	Caucasian		Asian
	Latino/Latina		Caucasian
			Latino/Latina

Faculty

Name			Highest Degree	Rank	Time	Credentials State Lic.	NCC	Email
Bradley	Fred	O	PhD	Full Professor		Y	Y	fbradley@ksu.edu
Carlstrom	Aaron	H	PhD	Assistant Professor	>81	N	N	acarlstr@ksu.edu
Harris	Brandonn		PhD	Assistant Professor			Y	bsharris@ksu.edu
Hughey	Judith	K	EdD	Associate Professor			Y	jhughey@ksu.edu
Hughey	Kenneth	F	PhD	Full Professor		Y	Y	khughey@ksu.edu
Jones	Carla	E	PhD	Assistant Professor	<21		N	cjones@ksu.edu
Moran	Christy		PhD	Associate Professor		N	N	cmoran@ksu.edu
Newton	Fred	B	PhD	Full Professor	22-40		N	newtonf@ksu.edu
Nutt	Charles	L	PhD	Assistant Professor			N	cnutt@ksu.edu
Wilcox	Dan		PhD	Assistant Professor			N	dwilcox@ksu.edu
Wright-Carrroll	Doris		PhD	Associate Professor	>81		Y	djwright@ksu.edu

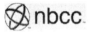 Percent of faculty with NCC certification: 45%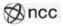

Other Credentials Held By Faculty Members: Licensed Psychologist, LPC Supervisor

Enrollment and Admission Requirements

Degree	Program	Gender F	M	Yearly Admit	Grad	GRE Total	MAT	Master	GPA	Work Exp	Letters	Interview
MS	Academic Advising	25	25	50	20			Y	3			N
Other	Academic Advising Certificate			50	50			Y	3			N
								Y	3			
MS	School Counseling	40	8	25	15	970	399	Y	3	1	3	
MS	Student Affairs	20	20	20	10	1000	399	Y	3		3	
MS	Student Services in Intercollegiate Athletics	10	10	20	10	1000	399				3	
PhD	Counselor Education	5	2	5	2	1000		Y	3	2	3	N
PhD	Student Affairs	8	6	6	4	1000		Y	3		3	

Graduation Requirements

Degree	Program	Academic Hours Sem	Qtr	Clock Hours Pract	Intern	Thesis	Comp	Examinations CPCE	Oral	Portfolio
MS	Academic Advising	30				N	N			Y
Other	Academic Advising Certificate	15				N	Y			
MS	School Counseling	48		100	600	N	Y			
MS	Student Affairs	39		50	160		Y			
MS	Student Services in Intercollegiate Athletics	39		50	160					
PhD	Counselor Education	120		100	600	Y	Y			
PhD	Student Affairs	93		50	160	Y	Y			

KS: Pittsburg State University

1701 S. Broadway
Pittsburg, KS 66762-7557
United States of America
www.pittstate.edu/department/psychology/programs-and-degrees/graduate-degree-programs.dot#CMH

Dean
Howard Smith
College of Education
Pittsburg, KS 66762
United States of America

Administrator
David P. Hurford, Chair
1701 S. Broadway
Pittsburg, KS 66762-7557
United States of America
(316) 235-4522; fax: (316) 235-4520
psych@pittstate.edu

CSI Chapter, Name   NP
Regionally Accredited   Y
Financial Aid   Y

Satellite Campus: N
International Students: Y
Number of International Students: 1

Program Uniqueness

The department offers an eclectic approach that is highly applied.

Faculty Research

Life-span development, family systems counseling, multicultural counseling, marriage counseling, clinical mental health counseling, group processes, group dynamics, group counseling, team building, theories and techniques of counseling and psychotherapy, cinematherapy, human sexuality, addictions counseling, integrative-eclectic models.

40% faculty in professional counseling practice.

Program Accreditation

CACREP: Community Counseling

Degree Programs

Degree	Program	Contact
MS	Clinical Mental Health Counseling	Donald Ward

M	School Counseling	Becky Brannock
EdS	Clinical Mental Health Counseling	Donald Ward
EdS	School Counseling	Becky Brannock

Distance learning: N; 0% courses on-line

Other Counseling Related Programs

Psychology

Faculty and Student Ethnicity

Faculty	**Master's**	**Specialist**	**Doctoral**
Caucasian	Caucasian	Caucasian	
Other	Latino/Latina		
	Native American		

Faculty

Name			Highest Degree	Rank	Time	Credentials State Lic.	NCC	Email
Bachner	Harriet	A	PhD	Assistant Professor	>81	Y	N	hbachner@pittstate.edu
Brannock	Becky	S	PhD	Professor	>81	Y	N	rbrannoc@pittstate.edu
Rush	Conni	K	EdD	Professor	>81	Y	Y	csharp@pittstate.edu
Spera	Chris	M	PhD	Assistant Professor	>81	N	N	cspera@pittstate.edu
Ward	Donald	E	PhD	Professor	>81	Y	Y	dward@pittstate.edu

 nbcc   Percent of faculty with NCC certification: 40%   **ncc**

Other Credentials Held By Faculty Members: AAMFT Clinical Member, Approved Clinical Supervisor, CCMHC, Certified School Counselor, LMFT, LPC

Enrollment and Admission Requirements

Degree	Program	Gender F	M	Yearly Admit	Grad	GRE Total	MAT	Master	GPA	Work Exp	Letters	Interview
MS	Clinical Mental Health Counseling	16	5	10	8	800		Y	3		3	N
M	School Counseling	22	12	12	10	800		Y	3		3	N
EdS	Clinical Mental Health Counseling			3	3			Y			3	N
EdS	School Counseling			3	3			Y			3	N

Graduation Requirements

Degree	Program	Academic Hours Sem	Qtr	Clock Hours Pract	Intern	Thesis	Comp	Examinations CPCE	Oral	Portfolio
MS	Clinical Mental Health Counseling	60		100	600	N	Y	N	N	N
M	School Counseling	48	41	150	150	N	Y	N	N	Y
EdS	Clinical Mental Health Counseling	32				N	Y	N	N	N
EdS	School Counseling	32				N	Y	N	N	

KY: Northern Kentucky University

BEP 203
Department of Counseling, Social Work, and Leadership
Highland Heights, KY 41099
United States of America
http://www.nku.edu/~ahhssw/

Dean

Mark Wascisko
College of Education and Human Services
BEP 224
Highland Heights, KY 41099
United States of America

Administrator

Larry Sexton, Chair and Professor
BEP 203
Highland Heights, KY 41099
United States of America
(859) 572-5604; fax: (859) 572-6592
sexton1@nku.edu

CSI Chapter, Name   Y, Nu Kappa
Regionally Accredited Y
Financial Aid   Y

Satellite Campus: N
International Students: Y
Number of International Students: 10

Program Uniqueness

An off-campus training and development center for interns that features supervision. This center is externally funded and supported by NKU and the justice system of Campbell County.

Faculty Research

NP

20% faculty in professional counseling practice.

Degree Programs

Degree	Program	Contact
MS	Clinical Mental Health Counseling	Jacqueline Smith, Ed.D.
MA	School Counseling	Brett Zyromski, Ph.D.

Distance learning: Y; 10% courses on-line

Other Counseling Related Programs
NP

Faculty and Student Ethnicity

Faculty	Master	Specialist	Doctoral
	African-American		
	Asian		
	Biracial		

Faculty

Name			Highest Degree	Rank	Time	State Lic.	NCC	Email
						Credentials		
Altekruse	Michael	K	EdD	Full Professor	61-80	N	Y	altekrusem1@nku.edu
Engebretson	Ken		PhD	Assistant Professor	61-80	Y	Y	engebretsk1@nku.edu
Hatchett	Greg		PhD	Associate Professor	61-80	Y	Y	hatchettg@nku.edu
Sexton	Larry		EdD	Professor and Chair	<21	Y	N	sextonl1@nku.edu
Smith	Jacqueline		EdD	Associate Professor and Director of Counselor Education	61-80	Y	N	smithjac@nku.edu
Wilkerson	David		MSW	Director of Counseling and Training Center		Y	N	wilkersond1@nku.edu
Zyromski	Brett		PhD	Assistant Professor	61-80	Y	Y	

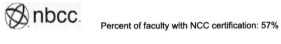

Percent of faculty with NCC certification: 57%

Other Credentials Held By Faculty Members: Certified Elementary School Counselor, Certified School Counselor, LPC, LSSW, LSW

Enrollment and Admission Requirements

Degree	Program	Gender		Yearly		GRE Total	MAT	Master	GPA	Work Exp	Letters	Interview
		F	M	Admit	Grad							
MS	Clinical Mental Health Counseling	40	20	20	10	0		Y		0	3	Y
MA	School Counseling	90	30	40	10	0		Y		0	3	

Graduation Requirements

Degree	Program	Academic Hours		Clock Hours				Examinations		
		Sem	Qtr	Pract	Intern	Thesis	Comp	CPCE	Oral	Portfolio
MS	Clinical Mental Health Counseling	60		100	600	N	N	Y	N	N
MA	School Counseling									

LA: Louisiana State University

122 Peabody Hall
Baton Rouge, LA 70803-4721
United States of America
http://coe.ednet.lsu.edu/coe/ETPP/counseling/counseling.html

Dean

Jayne Fleener
College of Education, 221 Peabody Hall
Baton Rouge, LA 70803-4721
United States of America

Administrator

Gary G. Gintner, PhD
Coordinator of Counselor Education and Associate Professor
122 Peabody Hall
Baton Rouge, LA 70803-4721
United States of America
(225) 578-2197; fax: NP
gintner@lsu.edu

CSI Chapter. Name NP
Regionally Accredited Y
Financial Aid Y

Satellite Campus: N
International Students: Y
Number of International Students: 2

Program Uniqueness

The program emphasizes close collaboration between students and faculty. There is a strong emphasis on evidence-based treatment approaches and practical in-class and out-of-class clinical experiences in each course.

Faculty Research

Gary G. Gintner, PhD.: designing effective treatment plans, practice guidelines for psychiatric disorders and effectiveness of motivational interviewing for substance use problems; David A. Spruill, PhD.: training issues in marriage and family counseling, professional development issues, and ethics; Laura G. Hensley, PhD.: women`s issues, sexual assault, college counseling, and group work.

100% faculty in professional counseling practice.

Program Accreditation

CACREP: Community Counseling; **CACREP:** School Counseling

Degree Programs

Degree	Program	Contact
M	Community Counseling	Laura G. Hensley, Ph.D.
M	School Counseling	Dr. Jennifer Curry
S	Community Counseling	Gary G. Gintner, Ph.D.
S	School Counseling	David A. Spruill, Ph.D.

Distance learning: N; 0% courses on-line

Other Counseling Related Programs

Clinical Social Workers
Communications
Psychology

Faculty and Student Ethnicity

Faculty	Master's	Specialist	Doctoral
Caucasian	African-American	African-American	
	Asian-American	Asian-American	
	Caucasian	Caucasian	

Faculty

Name			Highest Degree	Rank	Time	Credentials State Lic.	NCC	Email
Curry	Jennifer		PhD	Assistant Professor	41-60	N	N	jcurry@lsu.edu
Gintner	Gary	G	PhD	Associate Professor	41-60	Y	N	gintner@lsu.edu
Hensley	Laura	G	PhD	Associate Professor	41-60	Y	N	lhensley@lsu.edu

Percent of faculty with NCC certification: 0%

Other Credentials Held By Faculty Members: Approved Clinical Supervisor, Certified School Counselor, LPC, LPC Supervisor, NCSC

Enrollment and Admission Requirements

Degree	Program	Gender F	M	Yearly Admit	Grad	GRE Total	MAT	Master	GPA	Work Exp	Letters	Interview
M	Community Counseling	22	1	10	9	1000		Y	3		3	Y
M	School Counseling	7	1	8	5	0		Y	3		3	Y
S	Community Counseling	22	1	10	9	0					3	
S	School Counseling	10		5	5						3	

Graduation Requirements

Degree	Program	Academic Hours Sem	Qtr	Clock Hours Pract	Intern	Thesis	Comp	Examinations CPCE	Oral	Portfolio
M	Community Counseling	48		100	600	N	N	Y	N	N
M	School Counseling	48		100	600	N	N	Y	N	N
S	Community Counseling	60			300		Y			
S	School Counseling	60			300		Y			

LA: Our Lady of Holy Cross College

4123 Woodland Drive
New Orleans, LA 70131
United States of America
www.olhcc.edu

Dean NP

Administrator Carolyn C. White, Chair
4123 Woodland Drive
New Orleans, LA 70131
United States of America
(504) 398-2149; fax: (504) 398-2115
cwhite@olhcc.edu

CSI Chapter, Name Y, Alpha Zeta
Regionally Accredited Y
Financial Aid Y

Satellite Campus: N
International Students: N
Number of International Students: 0

Program Uniqueness
NP

Faculty Research
NP

100% faculty in professional counseling practice.

Program Accreditation

CACREP: Community Counseling; **CACREP:** Marital, Couple and Family
Counseling/Therapy; **CACREP:** School Counseling

Degree Programs

Degree	Program	Contact
MA	Community Counseling	Dr. Carolyn C. White
MA	Marriage, Couple, and Family Counseling	Dr. Carolyn C. White
MA	School Counseling	Dr. Carolyn C. White

Distance learning: N; 0% courses on-line

Other Counseling Related Programs: NP

Faculty and Student Ethnicity

Faculty	**Master's**	**Specialist**	**Doctoral**
Caucasian	African-American		
Latino/Latina	Asian-American		
	Caucasian		
	Latino/Latina		

Faculty

Name			Highest Degree	Rank	Time	Credentials State Lic.	NCC	Email
Fischer	Joan		MA	Director of Counseling and Training Center		Y	Y	jfischer@olhcc.edu
Hay	George	N	DMin	Associate Professor		Y	N	ghay@olhcc.edu
Morris	Matthew		PhD	Assistant Professor		Y	N	mmorris@olhcc.edu
Salgado	Roy		PhD	Assistant Professor		Y	N	rsalgado@olhcc.edu
White	Carolyn	C	PhD	Associate Professor and Chair		Y	Y	cwhite@olhcc.edu

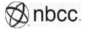 Percent of faculty with NCC certification: 40%

Other Credentials Held By Faculty Members: AAMFT Approved Supervisor, AAMFT Clinical Member, Approved Clinical Supervisor, LMFT, LPC, LPC Supervisor

Enrollment and Admission Requirements

Degree	Program	Gender F	M	Yearly Admit	Grad	GRE Total	MAT	Master	GPA	Work Exp	Letters	Interview
MA	Community Counseling			20	15	0		Y	3		3	Y
MA	Marriage, Couple, and Family Counseling			20	20			Y	3		3	Y
MA	School Counseling			15	10			Y	3		3	Y

Graduation Requirements

Degree	Program	Academic Hours Sem	Qtr	Clock Hours Pract	Intern	Thesis	Examinations Comp	CPCE	Oral	Portfolio
MA	Community Counseling	60		100	600	N	Y	Y	Y	N
MA	Marriage, Couple, and Family Counseling	60		100	600	N	Y	Y	Y	N
MA	School Counseling	60		100	600	N	Y	Y	Y	N

MD: Loyola University Maryland

8890 McGaw Road
Columbia, MD 21045
United States of America
www.Loyola.edu/pastoral

Dean   James Buckley, Dean
                  Loyola College of Arts and Sciences
                  Humanities Building
                  Baltimore, MD 21210
                  United States of America

Administrator   Sharon Cheston, Chair
                      8890 McGaw Road STE 380
                      Columbia, MD 21045
                      United States of America
                      (410) 617-7620; fax: (410) 617-7644
                      dcnewton@loyola.edu

CSI Chapter, Name   NP
Regionally Accredited Y
Financial Aid   Y

Satellite Campus: Y
International Students: Y
Number of International Students: 30

Program Uniqueness

The goal of the Master's of Science program is to develop competent practitioners of the counseling profession who give the spiritual dimension an integral role as they help others. Our M.S. students complete a rigorous academic and clinical program that meets the education requirements to eventually become licensed professional counselors. The Ph.D. program seeks to prepare graduates to become advanced practitioners and make research contributions to the helping professions through the integration of psycho-theological issues with counselor education's interdisciplinary models. Students in this program tend to become faculty members in counselor education graduate programs, researchers, or advanced practitioners, supervisors, and directors within clinical centers. The multicultural, racial and ethnic mix of the programs is well above the national average, with students and alumni representing all 50 states and more than 45 countries around the world. There is also great diversity in the faith traditions honored by the students and alumni within the programs—Catholic, Protestant, Jewish, Hindu, Buddhist, Muslim and other wisdom traditions. Together, the diversity of cultures and religious traditions add to the context and the richness of what the programs are meant to be.

Faculty Research

Counseling education, spirituality, resilience, research and treatment of psychopathology, clinical work with abused clients, addictions, personality, NEO, trauma and spirituality.

75% faculty in professional counseling practice.

Program Accreditation

CACREP: Community Counseling; **CACREP:** Counselor Education and Supervision

Degree Programs

Degree	*Program*	*Contact*
MS	Clinical Mental Health Counseling	Brenda Helsing
Post-master Certificate	Pastoral Counseling	Brenda Helsing
PhD	Pastoral Counseling	Brenda Helsing

Distance learning: N; % courses on-line: NP

Other Counseling Related Programs

Psychology
School Counseling
Spiritual and Pastoral Care

Faculty and Student Ethnicity

Faculty	**Master's**	**Specialist**	**Doctoral**
African-American	African-American	African-American	African-American
Caucasian	Asian-American	Asian-American	Asian
Pacific Islander	Caucasian	Caucasian	Multiracial
	Latino/Latina	Latino/Latina	Native American
	Multiracial	Multiracial	Other
	Native American	Native American	
	Pacific Islander	Other	

Faculty

Name			Highest Degree	Rank	Time	Credentials State Lic.	NCC	Email
Cheston	Sharon	E	EdD	Full Professor	>81		Y	SCheston@Loyola.edu
Ciarrocchi	Joseph	W	PhD	Full Professor	>81		N	JCiarrocchi@Loyola.edu
Fialkowski	Geraldine	M	PhD	Assistant Professor	>81		Y	GFialkowski@Loyola.edu
Jeffreys	Shep		EdD	Assistant Professor	22-40		N	JJeffreys@Loyola.edu
Lasure-Bryant	Danielle	R	EdD	Clinical Faculty	<21	Y	Y	drlasurebryant@loyola.edu
Magyar-Russell	Gina	M	PhD	Assistant Professor	>81	N	N	gmmagyarrussell@loyola.edu
McLaughlin	John	L	PhD	Assistant Professor	41-60		N	JMcLaughlin@Loyola.edu
Murray-Swank	Nichole	A	PhD	Assistant Professor		N	N	namurrayswak@loyola.edu
O'Grady	Kari	A	PhD	Assistant Professor		Y	Y	karogrady@loyola.edu
Oakes	Katherine	E	PhD	Assistant Professor	>81		N	KOakes@Loyola.edu
Piedmont	Ralph	L	PhD	Full Professor		N	N	RPiedmont@Loyola.edu
Rodgerson	Thomas		PhD	Assistant Professor	22-40	Y	Y	trodgerson@Loyola.edu
Stewart-Sicking	Joseph	A	PhD	Assistant Professor	>81	Y	N	jastewartsicking@loyola.edu
Wicks	Robert	J	PsyD	Full Professor	>81		N	RWicks@Loyola.edu

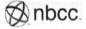   Percent of faculty with NCC certification: 36%

Other Credentials Held By Faculty Members: Approved Clinical Supervisor, Licensed Psychologist

Enrollment and Admission Requirements

Degree	Program	Gender		Yearly		GRE Total	MAT	Master	GPA	Work Exp	Letters	Interview
		F	M	Admit	Grad							
MS	Clinical Mental Health Counseling	75	25	60	60			Y			2	Y
Post-master Cert	Pastoral Counseling	75	25	20	20			Y			2	Y
PhD	Pastoral Counseling			12	10			Y		2	2	Y

Graduation Requirements

Degree	Program	Academic Hours		Clock Hours		Examinations				
		Sem	Qtr	Pract	Intern	Thesis	Comp	CPCE	Oral	Portfolio
MS	Clinical Mental Health Counseling	66			800	N	N	N	N	Y
Post-master Cert	Pastoral Counseling	30				N	N	N	N	N
PhD	Pastoral Counseling	60			600	Y	N	N	N	Y

ME: Husson University

1 College Circle
Bangor, ME 04401
United States of America
www.husson.edu

Dean   Barbara Higgins
College of Health and Education
O'Donnell Commons
Husson University
Bangor, ME 04401
United States of America

Administrator   Deborah L. Drew
Associate Professor and
Director of Programs in Counseling and Human Relations
312 Commons
Husson University
1 College Circle
Bangor, ME 04401
United States of America
(207) 992-4912; fax: (207) 992-4952
drewd@husson.edu

CSI Chapter, Name   N
Regionally Accredited Y
Financial Aid   Y

Satellite Campus: Y
International Students: N
Number of International Students: 0

Program Uniqueness

Offers Master of Science programs in school counseling, clinical mental health counseling, pastoral counseling and human relations in four locations in Maine.

Faculty Research

Rural counseling, ethics, self-care, and clinical supervision.

67% faculty in professional counseling practice.

Degree Programs

Degree	Program	Contact
MS	Clinical Mental Health Counseling	Dr. Deborah Drew
MS	Human Relations	Dr. Deborah Drew
MS	Pastoral Counseling	Dr. Deborah Drew
MS	School Counseling	Dr. Deborah Drew

Distance learning: Y; 5% courses on-line

Other Counseling Related Programs
NP

Faculty and Student Ethnicity

Faculty	**Master's**	**Specialist**	**Doctoral**
Caucasian	African-American		
	Caucasian		
	Latino/Latina		
	Multiracial		

Faculty

Name			Highest Degree	Rank	Time	Credentials State Lic.	NCC	Email
Crawford	Mikal		EdD	Associate Professor		N	Y	crawfordm@husson.edu
Drew	Deborah	L	EdD	Associate Professor and Director of Counselor Education		Y	Y	drewd@husson.edu
Stevens	Jeri	W	PhD		41-60	Y	Y	stevensj@fc.husson.edu

Percent of faculty with NCC certification: 100%

Other Credentials Held By Faculty Members: ACS, Approved Clinical Supervisor, CCMHC, Certified School Counselor, Licensed Psychologist, LPC

Enrollment and Admission Requirements

Degree	Program	Gender F M	Yearly Admit Grad	GRE Total	MAT	Master	GPA	Work Exp	Letters	Interview
MS	Clinical Mental Health Counseling			0		Y			3	Y
MS	Human Relations			0		Y			3	Y
MS	Pastoral Counseling			0		Y			3	Y
MS	School Counseling					Y			3	Y

Graduation Requirements

Degree	Program	Academic Hours Sem Qtr	Clock Hours Pract Intern		Examinations Thesis	Comp	CPCE	Oral	Portfolio
MS	Clinical Mental Health Counseling	61	100	900	N	Y	Y	N	N
MS	Human Relations	37			N	N	N	N	N
MS	Pastoral Counseling	57		400	N	N	Y	N	N
MS	School Counseling	40	120	600	N	N	N	N	Y

MI: Eastern Michigan University

304 Porter
Ypsilanti, MI 48197-2706
United States of America
www.emich.edu/coe/Lead_Coun/

Dean   Michael Bretting, Interim Dean
College of Education
Porter Building
Ypsilanti, MI 48197
United States of America

Administrator Jaclynn C. Tracy, Department Head
304 Porter
Ypsilanti, MI 48197-2706
United States of America
(734) 487-0255; fax: (734) 487-4608

CSI Chapter, Name   Y, Pi Omega
Regionally Accredited Y
Financial Aid   Y

Satellite Campus: N
International Students: Y
Number of International Students: NP

Program Uniqueness

State-of-the-art counseling clinic where students complete their counseling practicum. Post-master's certificate programs in multiculturalism and school counseling. Core courses offered at one off-campus location (Flint). Faculty maintain and encourage strong participation in professional organizations.

Faculty Research

Multicultural issues in counseling; supervision.

30% faculty in professional counseling practice.

Program Accreditation

CACREP: College Counseling; **CACREP:** Community Counseling; **CACREP:** School Counseling

Degree Programs

Degree	Program	Contact
MA	College Counseling	Perry Francis
MA	Community Counseling	Irene Ametrano
MA	School Counseling	Suzanne Dugger

Distance learning: N; 10% courses on-line

Other Counseling Related Programs

Clinical Social Workers
Communications
Psychology

Faculty and Student Ethnicity

Faculty	**Master's**	**Specialist**	**Doctoral**
African-American	African-American		
Caucasian	Asian-American		
Other	Caucasian		
	Latino/Latina		
	Multiracial		

Faculty

Name			Highest Degree	Rank	Time	Credentials State Lic.	NCC	Email
Ametrano	Irene	M	EdD	Full Professor	>81	Y	Y	iametrano@emich.edu
Callaway	Yvonne	L	PhD	Full Professor	>81	Y	N	ycallaway@emich.edu
Choudhuri	Devika	D	PhD	Associate Professor	>81	Y	Y	dibya.choudhuri@emich.edu
Dugger	Suzanne	M	EdD	Full Professor	>81	Y	N	sdugger@emich.edu
Francis	Perry		EdD	Full Professor	41-60	Y	Y	pfrancis@emich.edu
Parfitt	Diane	L	PhD	Associate Professor	>81	Y	N	dparfitt@emich.edu
Sticke	Sue	A	PhD	Full Professor		Y	N	sstickel@emich.edu

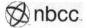 Percent of faculty with NCC certification: 43%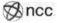

Other Credentials Held By Faculty Members: ACS

Enrollment and Admission Requirements

Degree	Program	Gender F	M	Yearly Admit	Grad	GRE Total	MAT	Master	GPA	Work Exp	Letters	Interview
MA	College Counseling	7	3	10	8	0		Y	2.75		3	Y
MA	Community Counseling	15	5	20	12	0		Y	2.75		3	Y
MA	School Counseling	40	10	50	35	0			2.75		3	Y

Graduation Requirements

Degree	Program	Academic Hours Sem	Qtr	Clock Hours Pract	Intern	Thesis	Comp	Examinations CPCE	Oral	Portfolio
MA	College Counseling	48		100	600	N	N	Y	N	N
MA	Community Counseling	48		100	600	N	N	Y	N	N
MA	School Counseling	48		100	600			Y		N

MI: Oakland University

School of Education and Human Services
Rochester, MI 48309
United States of America
http://www.oakland.edu/counseling/

Dean   William Kean, Interim Dean
                            School of Education and Human Services

Administrator   Lisa Hawley, Ph.D., Associate Professor and Chair
                            School of Education and Human Services
                            Rochester, MI 48309
                            United States of America
                            (248) 370-2841; fax: (248) 370-4141
                            hawley@oakland.edu

CSI Chapter, Name   NP
Regionally Accredited Y
Financial Aid   Y

Satellite Campus: N
International Students: Y
Number of International Students: 5

Program Uniqueness

State of the art clinical and classroom facilities, suburban location, growing campus, diverse faculty, advanced specializations in mental health counseling, child and adolescent counseling, advanced career counseling, couple and family counseling, and school counseling.

Faculty Research

Trauma, group counseling, socioeconomic status in counseling, technology and supervision, couples counseling, integration of psychoanalytic and humanist therapies, adult transition, career and multicultural issues.

75% faculty in professional counseling practice.

Program Accreditation

CACREP: Community Counseling; **CACREP:** Counselor Education and Supervision; **CACREP:** School Counseling

Degree Programs

Degree	Program	Contact
M	Community Counseling	Luellen Ramey
	School Counseling	Lisa Hawley
PhD	Career Counseling	Brian Taber
PhD	Community Counseling	Lisa Hawley
PhD	Counselor Education	Lisa Hawley
PhD	Marriage and Family Counseling	Elizabeth Cron or Thomas Blume
PhD	Mental Health Counseling	James T. Hansen
PhD	School Counseling	Lisa Hawley
PhD	Wellness Specialization	Ramey Luellen

Distance learning: N; 10% courses on-line

Other Counseling Related Programs

Psychology

Faculty and Student Ethnicity

Faculty	**Master's**	**Specialist**	**Doctoral**
Caucasian	African-American		African-American
	Asian-American		Asian
	Caucasian		Caucasian
	Latino/Latina		Latino/Latina
	Multiracial		

Faculty

Name			Highest Degree	Rank	Time	Credentials State Lic.	NCC	Email
Binkley	Erin		PhD	Assistant Professor	>81	N	N	binkley@oakland.edu
Blume	Thomas	W	PhD	Associate Professor	>81	Y	N	blume@oakland.edu
Chaney	Michael		PhD	Assistant Professor		Y	Y	chaney@oakland.edu
Cron	Elizabeth	A	PhD	Associate Professor	>81	Y	N	ecron@oakland.edu
Day	Mary	R	PhD	Assistant Professor		Y	N	mrday@oakland.edu
Fink	Robert	S	PhD	Associate Professor	>81		Y	fink@oakland.edu
Hansen	James	T	PhD	Associate Professor	>81	Y	N	jthansen@oakland.edu
Hawley	Lisa	D	PhD	Assistant Professor	>81	Y	N	hawley@oakland.edu
Leibert	Todd	W	PhD	Assistant Professor	>81	Y	N	leibert@oakland.edu
Ramey	Luellen		PhD	Associate Professor		Y	Y	ramey@oakland.edu
Smiley	Kristin		PhD	Visiting Assistant Professor	>81	Y	Y	kasmiley@oakland.edu
Taber	Brian		PhD	Assistant Professor	>81	Y	Y	taber@oakland.edu

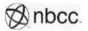 Percent of faculty with NCC certification: 42%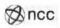

Other Credentials Held By Faculty Members: LMFT

Enrollment and Admission Requirements

Degree	Program	Gender F	M	Yearly Admit	Grad	GRE Total	MAT	Master	GPA	Work Exp	Letters	Interview
M	Community Counseling	61	9	85	70	0			3		2	Y
	School Counseling		8	75	60				3		2	Y
PhD	Career Counseling			1		0		Y	3		2	Y
PhD	Community Counseling			1		0		N	4		2	Y
PhD	Counselor Education			3	3	0		N	4		2	Y
PhD	Marriage and Family Counseling			1	1	0		N	4		2	Y
PhD	Mental Health Counseling			2		0		Y	3		2	Y
PhD	School Counseling					0		Y	3		2	Y
PhD	Wellness Specialization					0		Y	3			N

Graduation Requirements

Degree	Program	Academic Hours Sem	Qtr	Clock Hours Pract	Intern	Thesis	Comp	Examinations CPCE	Oral	Portfolio
M	Community Counseling	48		100	600					
	School Counseling	48		100	600					
PhD	Career Counseling	82		100	600	Y	Y			
PhD	Community Counseling	82		100	600	Y	Y			
PhD	Counselor Education	82		100	600	Y	Y			
PhD	Marriage and Family Counseling	82		100	600	Y	Y			
PhD	Mental Health Counseling	82		100	600	Y	Y			
PhD	School Counseling	82		100	600	Y				
PhD	Wellness Specialization									

MI: University of Detroit Mercy

4001 W. McNichols Rd.
Detroit, MI 48221
United States of America
www.udmercy.edu

Dean   Charles E. Marske
4001 W. McNichols Rd.
Detroit, MI 48221
United States of America

Administrator   NP

CSI Chapter, Name   N
Regionally Accredited Y
Financial Aid   Y

Satellite Campus: N
International Students: N
Number of International Students: 0

Program Uniqueness

Small, student-centered counseling program within a Jesuit institution in the city of Detroit. Class size is typically 10 students with small advisor caseloads to further promote a high degree of personal attention to each student. Social justice activism is a key part of the program as is service and advocacy within the urban environment providing us the appropriate context by which to promote a lifestyle of counselors as committed and fully engaged citizens.

Faculty Research
NP

% faculty in professional counseling practice: NP

Program Accreditation

CACREP

CACREP: Community Counseling; **CACREP:** School Counseling

Degree Programs
NP

Distance learning: N; 5% courses on-line

Other Counseling Related Programs
NP

Faculty and Student Ethnicity
NP

Faculty
NP

Percent of faculty with NCC certification: NP

Other Credentials Held By Faculty Members
NP

Enrollment and Admission Requirements
NP

Graduation Requirements
NP

MI: University of Phoenix

318 River Ridge Drive, NW
Grand Rapids, MI 49544
United States of America
www.phoenix.edu/westmichigan

Dean   College of Social Sciences
4605 E. Elwood Street
Phoenix, AZ 85040
United States of America

Administrator   Todd Peuler, Campus Director
318 River Ridge Drive, NW
Grand Rapids, MI 49544
United States of America
(616) 647-4831; fax: (616) 784-5300
Todd.Peuler@phoenix.edu

CSI Chapter, Name   N
Regionally Accredited Y
Financial Aid   Y

Satellite Campus: Y
International Students: Y
Number of International Students: NP

Program Uniqueness
NP

Faculty Research
NP

% faculty in professional counseling practice: NP

Degree Programs

Degree	*Program*	*Contact*
MS	Counseling	Julie Schaefer-Space

Distance learning: Y; 0% courses on-line

Other Counseling Related Programs
NP

Faculty and Student Ethnicity
NP

Faculty
NP

Percent of faculty with NCC certification: NP

Other Credentials Held By Faculty Members
NP

Enrollment and Admission Requirements

Degree	Program	Gender		Yearly		GRE	MAT	Master	GPA	Work	Letters	Interview
		F	M	Admit	Grad	Total				Exp		
MS	Counseling	8	2	30	10							

Graduation Requirements

Degree	Program	Academic Hours		Clock Hours			Examinations			
		Sem	Qtr	Pract	Intern	Thesis	Comp	CPCE	Oral	Portfolio
MS	Counseling									

MI: Western Michigan University

Department of Counselor Education and Counseling Psychology
3102 Sangren Hall
Kalamazoo, MI 49008
United States of America
http://www.wmich.edu/coe/cecp/

Dean
Gary Wegenke
College of Education and Human Development
3102 Sangren Hall
Department of Counselor Education and Counseling Psychology
Kalamazoo, MI 49008
United States of America

Administrator
Patrick H. Munley, Professor and Chair
3102 Sangren Hall
Department of Counselor Education and Counseling Psychology
Kalamazoo, MI 49008
United States of America
(269) 387-5100; fax: (269) 387-5090
patrick.munley@wmich.edu

CSI Chapter, Name   Y, Mu Beta
Regionally Accredited Y
Financial Aid   Y

Satellite Campus: NP
International Students: Y
Number of International Students: NP

Program Uniqueness

For the most current information, prospective students should visit our department website at
http://www.wmich.edu/coe/cecp/. The Counselor Education program at Western Michigan
University has been accredited by the Council for Accreditation of Counseling and Related
Educational Programs (CACREP) since 1983. Our doctoral program in counselor education is
racially diverse (25% African American). Primary focus of the doctoral program is to prepare
counseling professionals for the professorate. Academic Analytics recently published the third
edition of the Faculty Scholarly Productivity Index. The index is a ranking of graduate programs at
research universities based on per-capita scholarly accomplishments. Academic Analytics, a
private company owned in part by the State University of New York-Stony Brook, compiled the
data. It is based on the number of professors in a given program and the number of books and
journal articles they have written; the number of times other scholars have cited those
publications; and the awards, honors and grant dollars received. Counselor education at Western
Michigan University was ranked in the top 10 in the discipline nationally.

Faculty Research

Preparation of counselors in training, faculty development, child-rearing practices and parenting,
marriage and family therapy, clinical supervision, Adlerian counseling and its application to clinical
supervision, humanistic theory and the African American experience, and rehabilitation
counseling. For a detailed description of faculty research interests, please see our doctoral
program brochure, available for download at
http://www.wmich.edu/coe/cecp/forms/doc_brochure_ce.pdf

10% faculty in professional counseling practice.

Program Accreditation

CACREP: College Counseling; **CACREP:** Community Counseling; **CACREP:** Counselor Education and Supervision; **CACREP:** School Counseling; **CORE:** Rehabilitation Counseling

Degree Programs

Degree	Program	Contact
MA	Clinical Mental Health Counseling	Jennipher Wiebold
MA	College Counseling	
MA	Marriage, Couple and Family Counseling	
MA	Rehabilitation Counseling	
MA	School Counseling	
PhD	Counselor Education and Supervision	Dr. Stephen E. Craig

Distance learning: N; % courses on-line: 0%

Other Counseling Related Programs

Counseling Psychology (M.A. and Ph.D.)
Human Resources Development (M.A.)

Faculty and Student Ethnicity

Faculty	Master's	Specialist	Doctoral
African-American	African-American		African-American
Caucasian	Asian		Asian-American
	Asian-American		Biracial
	Caucasian		Caucasian
	Latino/Latina		Other
	Native American		

Faculty

Name			Highest Degree	Rank	Time	State Lic.	NCC	Email
Adkison-Bradley	Carla		PhD	Full Professor			N	
Anderson	Mary	L	PhD	Assistant Professor			Y	
Anderson	Mary	Z	PhD	Full Professor			N	
Andreadis	Nicholas		MD	Assistant Professor			N	
Bischof	Gary	H	PhD	Full Professor			N	
Buzas	Larry		Doctorate	Assistant Professor			N	
Craig	Stephen	E	PhD	Associate Professor and Director of Counselor Education			N	
Croteau	James		PhD	Full Professor			N	
Duncan	Lonnie	E	PhD	Associate Professor			N	
Hedstrom	Suzanne		EdD	Associate Professor			N	

Hovestadt	Alan		EdD	Full Professor	Y
Johnson	Phillip		PhD	Associate Professor	N
McDonnell	Kelly		PhD	Associate Professor	N
McLaughlin	Jerry		PhD	Assistant Professor	N
Morris	Joseph		PhD	Full Professor	N
Munley	Patrick	H	PhD	Chair	N
Sauer	Eric		PhD	Associate Professor	N
Wiebold	Jennipher		PhD	Associate Professor	N

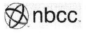   Percent of faculty with NCC certification: 11%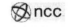

Other Credentials Held By Faculty Members
NP

Enrollment and Admission Requirements

Degree	Program	Gender F	M	Yearly Admit	Grad	GRE Total	MAT	Master	GPA	Work Exp	Letters	Interview
MA	Clinical Mental Health Counseling					0		Y			3	N
MA	College Counseling					0		Y			3	N
MA	Marriage, Couple and Family Counseling					0		Y			3	N
MA	Rehabilitation Counseling					0		Y			3	N
MA	School Counseling											
PhD	Counselor Education and Supervision							Y			3	Y

Graduation Requirements

Degree	Program	Academic Hours Sem	Qtr	Clock Hours Pract	Intern	Thesis	Comp	Examinations CPCE	Oral	Portfolio
MA	Clinical Mental Health Counseling	60		100	600	N	N	N	N	
MA	College Counseling	48		100	600	N	N	N	N	
MA	Marriage, Couple, and Family Counseling	60		100	600	N	N	N	N	
MA	Rehabilitation Counseling	48		100	600	N	N	N	N	
MA	School Counseling									
PhD	Counselor Education and Supervision	69				Y	Y	N	Y	

MN: Walden University

155 Fifth Avenue South, Suite 100
Minneapolis, MN 55401
United States of America
http://inside.waldenu.edu/c/Student_Faculty/StudentFaculty_4344.htm

Dean

Savitri Dixon-Saxon, Associate Dean
School of Counseling and Social Service
155 Fifth Avenue South, Suite 100
Minneapolis, MN 55401
United States of America

Administrator

Matthew R. Buckley
Program Director, M.S. in Mental Health Counseling
155 Fifth Avenue South, Suite 100
Minneapolis, MN 55401
United States of America
(800) 925-3368 ext 1443; fax: NP
matthew.buckley@waldenu.edu

CSI Chapter, Name   Y, Omega Zeta
Regionally Accredited   Y
Financial Aid   Y

Satellite Campus: Y
International Students: Y
Number of International Students: 20

Program Uniqueness

The M.S. in mental health counseling program is fully online and offers the advantages of quality distance learning. In addition to taking online courses, students participate in two mandatory, six-day residencies that are intensive learning formats designed to enhance classroom learning and professional development. The residency experience offers opportunities for community development and support, intensive skill building, group work, mentoring, supervision, advising and career planning. These academic residencies are prerequisites to practicum and internship.

Faculty Research
NP

50% faculty in professional counseling practice.

Program Accreditation

CACREP: Mental Health Counseling

Degree Programs
NP

Distance learning: Y; 100% courses on-line

Other Counseling Related Programs
NP

Faculty and Student Ethnicity

Faculty	Master's	Specialist	Doctoral
African-American	African-American		
Asian	Asian		
Caucasian	Asian-American		
Latino/Latina	Biracial		
Multiracial	Caucasian		
Other	Latino/Latina		
Pacific Islander	Multiracial		
	Native American		
	Other		
	Pacific Islander		

Faculty

Name			Highest Degree	Rank	Time	Credentials State Lic.	NCC	Email
Buckley	Matthew	R				Y	Y	matthew.buckley@waldenu.edu
Ford	Stephanie	JW	Doctorate	Full Professor and Director of the Master's Program	<21	Y	Y	stephanie.ford@waldenu.edu
Haight	Marilyn	G	Doctorate	Professor	41-60	Y	Y	marilyn.haight@waldenu.edu
Marszalek	John	F	Doctorate	Professor	41-60	Y	Y	john.marszalek@waldenu.edu
Milo	Lori	A	Doctorate	Professor	41-60	Y	N	lori.milo@waldenu.edu
Neswald-Potter	Rhonda		Doctorate	Professor	41-60	Y	N	rhonda.neswald-potter@waldenu.edu
Perepiczka	Michelle		Doctorate	Professor	41-60	Y	Y	michelle.perepiczka@waldenu.edu
Reicherzer	Stacee	L	Doctorate	Professor	61-80	Y	Y	stacee.reicherzer@waldenu.edu
Rush-Wilson	Tiffany	C	Doctorate	Professor	41-60	Y	Y	tiffany.rush-wilson@waldenu.edu
Sheperis	Donna		Doctorate	Professor	41-60	Y	Y	donna.sheperis@waldenu.edu
Strentzsch	Julie	A	Doctorate	Professor	61-80	Y	N	julie.strentzsch@waldenu.edu
Trippany	Robyn		Doctorate	Professor	61-80		N	robyn.trippany@waldenu.edu

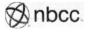 Percent of faculty with NCC certification: 67%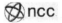

Other Credentials Held By Faculty Members: ACS, Approved Clinical Supervisor, Licensed Psychologist, LPC, LPC Supervisor, RPT

Enrollment and Admission Requirements
NP

Graduation Requirements
NP

MN: Winona State University

859 30th Ave. - S.E.
Rochester, MN 55904
United States of America
www.winona.edu/counselor education

Dean
Hank Rubin, College of Education
Winona State University, Gildemeister Hall 111
Winona, MN 55987
United States of America

Administrator
Gaylia Borror, Professor and Department Chair
859 30th Ave. - S.E.
Rochester, MN 55904
United States of America
(800) 366-5418, ext. 7137; fax: (507) 285-7170
www.winona.edu

CSI Chapter, Name Y, Rho Sigma Upsilon
Regionally Accredited Y
Financial Aid Y

Satellite Campus: Y
International Students: Y
Number of International Students: 2

Program Uniqueness

The goal of the Winona State University Counselor Education Department is to provide students with quality services and educational opportunities in order to help them meet their unique career goals. The Counselor Education Department is a student-friendly program that offers students support throughout their program of study. Employment upon graduation is high.

Faculty Research

Faculty members have a variety of research interests including play therapy, adolescent and infant mental health, marriage and family therapy, school counseling interventions, counseling college students, career counseling, multicultural counseling, and relationship skill development.

30% faculty in professional counseling practice.

Program Accreditation

 CACREP: Community Counseling; **CACREP:** School Counseling

Degree Programs

Degree	Program	Contact
MS	Community Counseling	Veronica Johnson
MS	Professional Development	Gaylia Borror
MS	School Counseling	Andrea Bjornestad
Advanced Graduate Certificate	Addictions Counseling Certificate Only	Gaylia Borror

Distance learning: Y; 20% courses on-line

Other Counseling Related Programs

Bachelor's in Psychology
Bachelor's in Social Work

Faculty and Student Ethnicity

Faculty	Master's	Specialist	Doctoral
Caucasian	African-American	Asian-American	
	Biracial	Biracial	
	Caucasian	Caucasian	
	Native American		

Faculty

Name		Highest Degree	Rank	Time	Credentials State Lic.	NCC	Email
Bjornestad	Andrea	PhD	Assistant Professor		N	Y	abjornestad@winona.edu
Borror	Gaylia	PhD	Professor		N	Y	gborror@winona.edu
Cigrand	Dawnette		Assistant Professor		N	N	dcigrand@winona.edu
Fawcett	Mary	PhD	Associate Professor		Y	Y	mfawcett@winona.edu
Hittner	Jo	PhD	Assistant Professor		Y	N	jhittner@winona.edu
Johnson	Veronica I	EdD	Assistant Professor		Y	Y	vjohnson@winona.edu

  Percent of faculty with NCC certification: 67%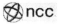

Other Credentials Held By Faculty Members: Licensed Psychologist, LPC, LPC Supervisor

Enrollment and Admission Requirements

Degree	Program	Gender F	M	Yearly Admit	Grad	GRE Total	MAT	Master	GPA	Work Exp	Letters	Interview
MS	Community Counseling	15	5	20	10	0		Y			3	Y
MS	Professional Development	8	2	10	5	0		Y	2.5		3	Y
MS	School Counseling	15	10	25	10	0		Y	2.5		3	Y
Advanced Graduate Certificate	Addictions Counseling Certificate Only	10	10	20	5	0		N				N

Graduation Requirements

Degree	Program	Academic Hours Sem	Qtr	Clock Hours Pract	Intern	Thesis	Examinations Comp	CPCE	Oral	Portfolio
MS	Community Counseling	48		150	600	N	Y	Y	N	Y
MS	Professional Development	34		0	0	N	Y	Y	N	Y
MS	School Counseling	48		150	600	N	Y	Y	N	Y
Advanced Graduate Certificate	Addictions Counseling Certificate Only	18			880	N	N	N	N	N

MO: University of Central Missouri

Lovinger 4101
Warrensburg, MO 64093
United States of America

Dean   NP

Administrator   NP

CSI Chapter, Name   NP
Regionally Accredited NP
Financial Aid   NP

Satellite Campus: NP
International Students: NP
Number of International Students: NP

Program Uniqueness
NP

Faculty Research
NP

% faculty in professional counseling practice: NP

Program Accreditation

CACREP: Community Counseling; **CACREP**: School Counseling

Degree Programs
NP

Distance learning: NP; % courses on-line: NP

Other Counseling Related Programs
NP

Faculty and Student Ethnicity
NP

Faculty
NP

Percent of faculty with NCC certification: NP

Other Credentials Held By Faculty Members
NP

Enrollment and Admission Requirements
NP

Graduation Requirements
NP

NC: Appalachian State University

Boone, NC 28608
United States of America

Dean NP

Administrator Lee Baruth, Chair
Boone, NC 28608
United States of America
(828) 262-2055; fax: (828) 262-2128
BaruthLG@appstate.edu

CSI Chapter, Name NP
Regionally Accredited Y
Financial Aid Y

Satellite Campus: N
International Students: Y
Number of International Students: 2

Program Uniqueness

High percentage of full-time students. Very student-oriented, student/practioner focus with emphasis on faculty as professional mentors.

Faculty Research
NP

% faculty in professional counseling practice: NP

Program Accreditation

CACREP: Community Counseling; **CACREP:** School Counseling

Degree Programs

Degree	*Program*	*Contact*
M	Clinical Mental Health Counseling	Keith Davis
M	Marriage and Family Counseling	Jon Winek
M	School Counseling	Laurie Williamson
M	Student Affairs	Cathy Clark

Distance learning: N; 0% courses on-line

Other Counseling Related Programs

Psychology

Faculty and Student Ethnicity

Faculty	Master's	Specialist	Doctoral
African-American	African-American		
Caucasian	Asian-American		
Native American	Caucasian		
	Latino/Latina		
	Native American		

Faculty

Name		Highest Degree	Rank	Time	Credentials State Lic.	NCC	Email
Atkins	Sally	EdD	Full Professor	>81		N	
Baruth	Lee	EdD	Full Professor	>81		N	
Caldwell	Karen	PhD	Associate Professor	>81	Y	N	
Clark	Cathy	PhD	Associate Professor	>81		N	
Davis	Keith	PhD	Full Professor			Y	
Ersever	Hakan	PhD	Assistant Professor	>81		N	
Evans	Renee'	PhD	Assistant Professor	>81	Y	N	
Galvin	Christina	PhD	Assistant Professor	>81	Y	N	
Lancaster	James	PhD	Assistant Professor	>81		N	
Miller	Geri	PhD	Full Professor	>81		N	
Mulgrew	Jack	PhD	Full Professor	>81		N	
Rodriguez	Chris	MA	Instructor	>81		N	
Scarboro	Barbara	PhD	Assistant Professor	>81	Y	Y	
Waryold	Diane	PhD	Associate Professor			N	
Williamson	Laurie	PhD	Full Professor	>81		Y	
Winek	Jon	PhD	Full Professor	>81		N	

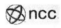 nbcc.   Percent of faculty with NCC certification: 19%   ncc

Other Credentials Held By Faculty Members: AAMFT Approved Supervisor, AAMFT Clinical Member

Enrollment and Admission Requirements

Degree	Program	Gender F	Gender M	Yearly Admit	Yearly Grad	GRE Total	MAT	Master	GPA	Work Exp	Letters	Interview
M	Clinical Mental Health Counseling			25	20						3	Y
M	Marriage and Family Counseling			12	11						3	Y
M	School Counseling			20	17						3	
M	Student Affairs			15	13						3	

Graduation Requirements

Degree	Program	Academic Hours Sem	Qtr	Clock Hours Pract	Clock Hours Intern	Thesis	Comp	CPCE	Oral	Portfolio
M	Clinical Mental Health Counseling	60		100	600		Y	Y		
M	Marriage and Family Counseling	48			500					
M	School Counseling	48		100	600		Y	Y		
M	Student Affairs	48		100	600					

NC: East Carolina University

Ragsdale Hall 213
Greenville, NC 27858
United States of America
http://www.ecu.edu/cs-educ/coad/Index.cfm

Dean

Linda Patriarcha
College of Education
154 Speight
Greenville, NC 27858
United States of America

Administrator

Vivian Mott, Department Chair
Ragsdale Hall 213
Greenville, NC 27858
United States of America
(252) 328-6856; fax: (252) 328-5114
mottv@ecu.edu

CSI Chapter, Name   NP
Regionally Accredited   Y
Financial Aid   Y

Satellite Campus: Y
International Students: Y
Number of International Students: 2

Program Uniqueness

The counselor education program provides a student-friendly curriculum with flexible elective study. Career options include school, agency and higher education.

Faculty Research

School counseling program evaluation, assessment in counseling, adventure based counseling, family counseling, diversity issues, career counseling.

% faculty in professional counseling practice: NP

Distance learning: Y; 33% courses on-line

Degree Programs

Degree	Program	Contact
M	Other	
S	Other	

Other Counseling Related Programs

Clinical Social Workers
Communications
Marriage and Family Therapists
Other
Psychiatric Nurses
Psychiatrists
Psychology

Faculty and Student Ethnicity

Faculty	Master's	Specialist	Doctoral
Caucasian	African-American	African-American	
	Caucasian	Caucasian	
	Latino/Latina	Latino/Latina	
	Native American	Native American	

Faculty

Name			Highest Degree	Rank	Time	Credentials State Lic.	NCC	Email
Ciechalski	Joseph	C	EdD	Full Professor	>81	Y	Y	ciechalskij@mail.ecu.edu
Dotson-Blake	Kylie		PhD	Assistant Professor	>81	Y	Y	blakek@ecu.edu
Glass	Scott		PhD	Associate Professor	>81	Y	Y	glassj@ecu.edu
Scholl	Mark		PhD	Assistant Professor	>81	N	Y	schollm@ecu.edu
Weaver	Florence	S	PhD	Full Professor	>81	Y	Y	weaverf@mail.ecu.edu

Percent of faculty with NCC certification: 100%

Other Credentials Held By Faculty Members
NP

Enrollment and Admission Requirements

Degree	Program	Gender F	M	Yearly Admit	Grad	GRE Total	MAT	Master	GPA	Work Exp	Letters	Interview
M	Other	1		40	28	1350	40		2.5		3	Y
S	Other	32	8	40	28		40				3	Y

Graduation Requirements

Degree	Program	Academic Hours Sem	Qtr	Clock Hours Pract	Intern	Thesis	Comp	Examinations CPCE	Oral	Portfolio
M	Other	48		90	225					
S	Other	30					Y			

NC: Gordon-Conwell Theological Seminary - Charlotte

14542 Choate Circle
Charlotte, NC 28273
United States of America

Dean Tim Laniak
Gordon Conwell Theological Seminary - Charlotte
14542 Choate Circle
Charlotte, NC 28273
United States of America

Administrator Maria L Boccia, Director
Gordon Conwell Theological Seminary - Charlotte
14542 Choate Circle
Charlotte, NC 28273
United States of America
(704) 527-9909; fax: (704) 527-8577
mboccia@gcts.edu

CSI Chapter, Name N
Regionally Accredited NP
Financial Aid Y

Satellite Campus: Y
International Students: Y
Number of International Students: NP

Program Uniqueness
NP

Faculty Research
NP

% faculty in professional counseling practice: NP

Program Accreditation
NP

Degree Programs
NP

Distance learning: Y; 33% courses on-line

Other Counseling Related Programs
NP

Faculty and Student Ethnicity
NP

Faculty
NP

Percent of faculty with NCC certification: NP

Other Credentials Held By Faculty Members
NP

Enrollment and Admission Requirements
NP

Graduation Requirements
NP

NC: North Carolina A&T State University

323 Proctor Hall 1601
East Market Street
Greensboro, NC 27411-1066
United States of America
www.ncat.edu

Dean   Ceola Ross Baber
School of Education
Proctor Hall
NC A&T State University
Greensboro, NC 27411-1066

Administrator   Miriam L. Wagner, Chairperson
323 Proctor Hall
1601 East Market Street
Greensboro, NC 27411-1066
United States of America
(336) 334-7916; fax: (336) 334-7280
wagnerm@ncat.edu

CSI Chapter, Name   Y, Alpha Tau Omega
Regionally Accredited Y
Financial Aid   Y

Satellite Campus: N
International Students: N
Number of International Students: 0

Program Uniqueness

Community and school counseling programs accredited by Council for Accreditation of Counseling and Related Programs (CACREP). Rehabilitation Counseling Programs accredited by CORE. Primarily an evening program.

Faculty Research

Grief and loss; assessment/evaluation; personality disorders; professional standards and practice; DSM-IV-TR criteria; spirituality; school counseling; addictions; vocational rehabilitation; workplace adjustment; behavior modification; college preparation; family counseling; diversity/multicultural issues.

% faculty in professional counseling practice: NP

Program Accreditation

CACREP: Community Counseling; **CACREP:** School Counseling; **CORE:** Rehabilitation Counseling

Degree Programs

Degree	Program	Contact
MS	Community Counseling	Dr. Patricia Bethea Whitfield
MS	Rehabilitation Counseling	Dr. Tyra T. Whittaker
MS	School Counseling	Dr. Shirlene Smith Augustine

Distance learning: Y; 10% courses on-line

Other Counseling Related Programs

Clinical Social Workers
Communications
International Studies
Marriage and Family Therapists
Psychology

Faculty and Student Ethnicity

Faculty	Master's	Specialist	Doctoral
African-American	African-American		
Caucasian	Caucasian		

Faculty

Name			Highest Degree	Rank	Time	State Lic.	NCC	Email
Bethea Whitfield	Patricia		EdD	Associate Professor	61-80		N	betheap@ncat.edu
Blalock	Kacie	M	PhD	Associate Professor	>81		N	kmblaloc@ncat.edu
Booth	Caroline		PhD	Assistant Professor		Y	Y	csbooth@ncat.edu
Boston	Quintin		PhD	Assistant Professor	>81		N	qboston@ncat.edu
Liles	Robin	G	PhD	Associate Professor		Y	Y	rgliles@ncat.edu
Lundberg	David		PhD	Associate Professor			Y	lundberg@ncat.edu
Lusk	Stephanie	L.	PhD	Assistant Professor			N	sllusk@ncat.edu
Smith Augustine	Shirlene		PhD	Assistant Professor			Y	saugusti@ncat.edu
Wagner	Miriam	L	EdD	Associate Professor	22-40		Y	wagnerm@ncat.edu
Webb	Tammy		PhD	Associate Professor			N	ttwebb@ncat.edu
Whittaker	Tyra	T	PhD	Associate Professor		Y	N	tnwhitta@ncat.edu

(Credentials)

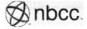 Percent of faculty with NCC certification: 45%

Other Credentials Held By Faculty Members: CRC, Licensed School Counselor, LSW, NCSC

Enrollment and Admission Requirements

Degree	Program	Gender F M	Yearly Admit Grad	GRE Total	MAT	Master	GPA	Work Exp	Letters	Interview
MS	Community Counseling			0		Y	3		3	Y
MS	Rehabilitation Counseling			0		Y	3		3	Y
MS	School Counseling			0		Y	3		3	Y

Graduation Requirements

Degree	Program	Academic Hours Sem Qtr	Clock Hours Pract	Intern	Thesis	Comp	CPCE	Oral	Portfolio
MS	Community Counseling	60	100	600	N	Y	Y	N	N
MS	Rehabilitation Counseling	48	100	600	N	Y	Y	N	N
MS	School Counseling	60	100	600	N	Y	Y	N	N

NC: North Carolina Central University

School of Education
712 Cecil Street
Durham, NC 27707
United States of America
www.nccuCounseling.com

Dean   Cecelia Steppe-Jones
Dean of the School of Education
School of Education, 712 Cecil Street
Durham, NC 27707
United States of America

Administrator   Edward E. Moody, Jr.
Professor and Chair of the Department of Counselor Education
School of Education, 712 Cecil Street
Durham, NC 27707
United States of America
(919) 530-5180; fax: (919) 530-5328
emoody@nccu.edu

CSI Chapter, Name   Y, Nu Chi Chi
Regionally Accredited Y
Financial Aid   Y

Satellite Campus: N
International Students: N
Number of International Students: 0

Program Uniqueness

We have a diverse student body. Students may pursue the program on a part- or full-time basis. Classes meet one day a week (4-6:30 pm or 7-9:30 pm), allowing students to work while pursuing their degree.

Faculty Research

Grief, trauma and substance abuse.

67% faculty in professional counseling practice.

Program Accreditation

CACREP: Career Counseling; **CACREP:** Community Counseling; **CACREP:** School Counseling

CACREP

Degree Programs

Degree	Program	Contact
MA	Career Counseling	Edward E. Moody, Jr.
MA	Community Counseling	Edward E. Moody, Jr.
MA	School Counseling	Edward E. Moody, Jr.

Distance learning: Y; 20% courses on-line

Other Counseling Related Programs: NP

Faculty and Student Ethnicity

Faculty	**Master's**	**Specialist**	**Doctoral**
African-American	African-American		
Caucasian	Caucasian		
	Latino/Latina		
	Multiracial		
	Native American		

Faculty

Name			Highest Degree	Rank	Time	Credentials State Lic.	NCC	Email
Kurian	Kyla		PhD	Assistant Professor	61-80	Y	Y	kkurian@nccu.edu
Lawrence	William		PhD	Full Professor	61-80	Y	Y	wlawrence@nccu.edu
Moody	Edward	E	PhD	Full Professor and Director of Graduate Program	22-40	Y	Y	emoody@nccu.edu
Newsome	Gwendolyn		PhD	Assistant Professor	61-80	Y	Y	gnewsome@nccu.edu
Royal	Chadwick		PhD	Assistant Professor	61-80	Y	Y	croyal@nccu.edu
Whiting	Peggy		EdD	Full Professor	61-80	Y	Y	pwhiting@nccu.edu

 nbcc   Percent of faculty with NCC certification: 100%   ncc

Other Credentials Held By Faculty Members: ACS, Licensed School Counselor, LPC, LPE

Enrollment and Admission Requirements

Degree	Program	Gender F	M	Yearly Admit	Grad	GRE Total	MAT	Master	GPA	Work Exp	Letters	Interview
MA	Career Counseling	9	5	7	7	800		Y	3	0	2	Y
MA	Community Counseling	12	3	15	15	800		Y	3	0	2	Y
MA	School Counseling	12	3	15	15	800		Y	3	0	2	Y

Graduation Requirements

Degree	Program	Academic Hours Sem	Qtr	Clock Hours Pract	Intern	Thesis	Examinations Comp	CPCE	Oral	Portfolio
MA	Career Counseling	48		100	600	N	Y	Y	N	Y
MA	Community Counseling	60		100	600	N	Y	Y	N	Y
MA	School Counseling	51		100	600	N	Y	Y	N	Y

NC: The University of North Carolina at Chapel Hill

Box #3500 - SOE
Chapel Hill, NC 27599
United States of America
http://soe.unc.edu/academics/med_sch_counseling/

Dean   NP

Administrator   NP

CSI Chapter, Name   N
Regionally Accredited   Y
Financial Aid   Y

Satellite Campus: N
International Students: Y
Number of International Students: 3

Program Uniqueness
NP

Faculty Research
NP

% faculty in professional counseling practice: NP

Program Accreditation

CACREP: School Counseling

Degree Programs
NP

Distance learning: N; 0% courses on-line

Other Counseling Related Programs
NP

Faculty and Student Ethnicity
NP

Faculty
NP

Percent of faculty with NCC certification: NP

Other Credentials Held By Faculty Members
NP

Enrollment and Admission Requirements
NP

Graduation Requirements
NP

NC: The University of North Carolina at Greensboro

P.O. Box 26170
Greensboro, NC 27402-6170
United States of America
www.uncg.edu/ced

Dean
Dale Schunk
School of Education

Administrator
J. Scott Young, Professor and Chair
PO Box 26170
Greensboro, NC 27402-6170
United States of America
(336) 334-3464; fax: (336) 334-3433
ced@uncg.edu

CSI Chapter, Name Y, Upsilon Nu Chi
Regionally Accredited Y
Financial Aid Y

Satellite Campus: N
International Students: Y
Number of International Students: NP

Program Uniqueness

Fulltime cohorts contribute to strong sense of community and shared learning. Supervised experience with clients throughout the program in state-of-the-art in-house clinic as well as field-based experiences. Five CACREP-accredited tracks at the master's level with options for Ed.S. also. CACREP-accredited doctoral program emphasizes advanced clinical skills, supervised teaching and supervision experiences, as well as strong research training. Faculty members are active researchers, quite involved in professional leadership, and provide active and deliberate mentoring of leadership skills for students. Program affiliates include Chi Sigma Iota and New Pathways Career Resource Center (state-wide, online) for high school students. Graduate assistantships and waivers are available.

Faculty Research

Career development/choice of adolescent females, particularly in math, science and engineering; peer supervision and consultation, clinical supervision process, supervisor training; adopted children and their families; violence prevention in the schools; substance abuse counseling; college student drinking behaviors and effective counseling interventions; play therapy; spiritual development; wellness and assessment of wellness; crisis intervention; cultural influences in academic achievement; professional issues (e.g., counselor credentialing, advocacy, ethics, women in nontraditional careers, gender role conflict, adolescent sex offenders, school counseling).

25% faculty in professional counseling practice.

Program Accreditation

CACREP: Counselor Education and Supervision; **CACREP:** Clinical Mental Health Counseling; **CACREP:** Marital, Couple, and Family Counseling; **CACREP:** School Counseling **CACREP:** Student Affairs

Degree Programs

Degree	*Program*
M	Clinical Mental Health Counseling
M	College Counseling and Student Development
M	Marriage, Couple, and Family Counseling
M	School Counseling
S	Community Counseling
S	Gerontological Counseling
S	Marriage and Family Counseling
S	School Counseling
S	Student Affairs
PhD	Counselor Education

Contact
For all programs in all tracks contact the Departmental admissions office at ced@uncg.edu or (336) 334-3434.

Distance learning: N; 5% courses on-line

Other Counseling Related Programs

Other
Psychiatric Nurses
Psychology

Faculty and Student Ethnicity

Faculty	**Master's**	**Specialist**	**Doctoral**
Caucasian	African-American	African-American	African-American
Latino/Latina	Asian-American	Asian-American	Asian
	Caucasian	Caucasian	Caucasian
	Latino/Latina	Latino/Latina	Latino/Latina
	Multiracial	Multiracial	Native American
	Native American	Native American	
	Pacific Islander	Other	

Faculty

Name			Highest Degree	Rank	Time	Credentials State Lic.	NCC	Email
Benshoff	James	M	PhD	Full Professor		Y	Y	benshoff@uncg.edeu
Borders	L. DiAnne		PhD	Full Professor		Y	Y	borders@uncg.edu
Cashwell	Craig	S	PhD	Full Professor		Y	Y	cscashwell@uncg.edu
Gonzalez	Laura		PhD	Assistant Professor		N	Y	lmgonza2@uncg.edu
Lewis	Todd		PhD	Associate Professor		Y	Y	tflewis@uncg.edu
Mobley	Keith		PhD	Associate Professor		Y	Y	akmobley@uncg.edu
Murray	Christine		PhD	Assistant Professor		Y	Y	cemurray@uncg.edu
Myers	Jane	E	PhD	Full Professor		Y	Y	jemyers@uncg.edu
Villalba	Jose	A	PhD	Associate Professor			Y	javillal@uncg.edu
Wester	Kelly	L	PhD	Associate Professor		Y	Y	klwester@uncg.edu
Young	J.	S	PhD	Chair		Y	Y	jsyoung3@uncg.edu

nbcc

Percent of faculty with NCC certification: 100%

ncc

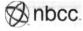

Other Credentials Held By Faculty Members: AAMFT Clinical Member, ACS, LMFT, LPC

Enrollment and Admission Requirements

Degree	Program	Gender		Yearly		GRE	MAT	Master	GPA	Work	Letters	Interview
		F	M	Admit	Grad	Total				Exp		
M	Clinical Mental Health Counseling	18	6	12	12	0			3		3	
M	College Counseling and Student Development	7	3	5	5	0			3		3	
M	Marriage, Couple and Family Counseling					0						
M	School Counseling	21	3	12	12	0			3		3	
S	Community Counseling	18	6	12	12	1000					3	
S	Gerontological Counseling	2	4	2	2						3	
S	Marriage and Family Counseling	4	3	8	8						3	
S	School Counseling	21	3	10	12						3	
S	Student Affairs	7		5	5						3	
PhD	Counselor Education			8	8			Y	3		3	Y

Graduation Requirements

Degree	Program	Academic Hours		Clock Hours		Examinations				
		Sem	Qtr	Pract	Intern	Thesis	Comp	CPCE	Oral	Portfolio
M	Clinical Mental Health Counseling	48		120	600	N	Y	N	N	
M	College Counseling and Student Development	48		120	600		Y			
M	Marriage, Couple and Family Counseling	48		120	600		Y			
M	School Counseling	48		120	600		Y			
S	Community Counseling	66		120	600		Y			
S	Gerontological Counseling	66		120	600		Y			
S	Marriage and Family Counseling	66		120	600		Y			
S	School Counseling	66		120	600		Y			
S	Student Affairs	66		120	600		Y			
PhD	Counselor Education	60		100	600	Y	Y		Y	

NC: University of North Carolina at Pembroke

PO Box 1510
Pembroke, NC 28372-1510
United States of America

Dean   NP

Administrator   NP

CSI Chapter, Name   NP
Regionally Accredited NP
Financial Aid   NP

Satellite Campus: NP
International students: NP
Number of International students: NP

Program Uniqueness
NP

Faculty Research
NP

        % faculty in professional counseling practice: NP

Degree Programs
NP

Distance learning: NP; % courses on-line: NP

Other Counseling Related Programs
NP

Faculty and Student Ethnicity
NP

Faculty
NP

Percent of faculty with NCC certification: NP

Other Credentials Held By Faculty Members
NP

Enrollment and Admission Requirements
NP

Graduation Requirements
NP

NC: Wake Forest University

Box 7406
Winston-Salem, NC 27109-7266
United States of America
www.wfu.edu/counseling

Dean

Lorna Moore
Graduate School of Arts and Sciences
Winston-Salem, NC 27109
United States of America

Administrator

Samuel T. Gladding, Chair
Department of Counseling
Box 7406
Winston-Salem, NC 27109-7266
United States of America
(336) 758-4932; fax: (336) 758-3129
karrpr@wfu.edu

CSI Chapter, Name   Y, Pi Alpha
Regionally Accredited   Y
Financial Aid   Y

Satellite Campus: N
International Students: N
Number of International Students: 0

Program Uniqueness

Small size allows much faculty/student interaction and strong cohort support. Partial tuition scholarships covering 85% of the cost are available to students.

Faculty Research

Samuel Gladding: creative arts and counseling, impact of lyrics; group counseling; counselors who worked with victims of 911. Donna Henderson: school counseling; counseling children; family counseling in schools. Debbie Newsome: girl's career-related interests in science, math and technology; expressive arts in counseling and supervision; counseling with children and adolescents. Edward Shaw: Grief counseling; Hospice; Alzheimers. Phillip Clarke: Spirituality; wellness; substance abuse. José Villalba: Latino and multicultural; wellness; school counseling.

60% faculty in professional counseling practice.

Program Accreditation

CACREP: Clinical Mental Health Counseling; **CACREP:** School Counseling

Degree Programs

Degree	Program	Contact
MA	Clinical Mental Health Counseling	Debbie Newsome
M	School Counseling	Donna A. Henderson

Distance learning : N; % courses on-line

Other Counseling Related Programs: NP

Faculty and Student Ethnicity

Faculty	Master's	Specialist	Doctoral
	African-American		
	Asian-American		
	Caucasian		
	Latino/Latina		
	Multiracial		

Faculty

Name			Highest Degree	Rank	Time	Credentials State Lic.	NCC	Email
Gladding	Samuel	T	PhD	Full Professor	>81	Y	Y	stg@wfu.edu
Henderson	Donna	A	PhD	Full Professor	>81	Y	Y	henderda@wfu.edu
Anderson	John	P	PhD	Full Professor	>81	Y	Y	jpa@wfu.edu
Newsome	Debbie		PhD	Associate Professor	>81	Y	Y	newsomdw@wfu.edu
Clarke	Phillip		PhD	Assistant Professor	>81	Y	Y	clarkpb@wfu.edu
Shaw	Edward		MD	Full Professor	22-40	N	Y	eshaw@wfubmc.edu
Villalba	José		PhD	Associate Professor	>81	Y	Y	villalb@wfu.edu

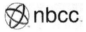 nbcc.   Percent of faculty with NCC certification: 100%   ncc

Other Certifications Held By Faculty Members: CC   MHC, NC Licensed K-12 School Counselor, LPC, ACS

Enrollment and Admission Requirements

Degree	Program	Gender F	M	Yearly Admit	Grad	GRE Total	MAT	Master	GPA	Work Exp	Letters	Interview
MA	Clinical Mental Health Counseling	7	4	9	9	1100		Y	3		3	Y
M	School Counseling	7	2	6	6	1100		Y	3		3	Y

Graduation Requirements

Degree	Program	Academic Hours Sem	Qtr	Clock Hours Pract	Intern	Thesis	Comp	Examinations CPCE	Oral	Portfolio
MA	Clinical Mental Health Counseling	60		200	600	N	Y	Y		Y
M	School Counseling	60		200	600	N	Y	Y		Y

ND: North Dakota State University

SGC C115
P.O. Box 6050
Fargo, ND 58105-6050
United States of America
www.ndsu.edu/ndsu/education/counselor_education/

Dean
Virginia Clark Johnson
College of Human Development and Education
EML 255
Fargo, ND 58105
United States of America

Administrator
William Martin, Head
Family Life Center, Room 210
Fargo, ND 58105-5057
United States of America
(701) 231-7202; fax: (701) 231-7416
William.Martin@ndsu.edu

CSI Chapter, Name   Y, Nu Delta Sigma
Regionally Accredited   Y
Financial Aid   Y

Satellite Campus: N
International Students: Y
Number of International Students: 2

Program Uniqueness

Only CACREP program in North Dakota.

Faculty Research

The person-centered approach; school counseling; stress management; cognitive/behavioral counseling; clinical mental health; multicultural counseling; professional ethics; qualitative research; career education; crisis management preparation; trauma; counselor education; counselor supervision; brief, solution-focused approaches; narrative therapy; intimate partner violence; collaborative practices; women as faculty members.

0% faculty in professional counseling practice.

Program Accreditation

CACREP: Community Counseling; **CACREP:** Counselor Education and Supervision; **CACREP:** School Counseling

Degree Programs

Degree	Program	Contact
MEd	Community Counseling	Jill R. Nelson
MEd	School Counseling	Carol B. Hoheisel
PhD	Counselor Education	Brenda S. Hall

Distance learning: Y; 5% courses on-line

Other Counseling Related Programs
NP

Faculty and Student Ethnicity

Faculty	Master's	Specialist	Doctoral
Native American	Native American		Native American

Faculty

Name			Highest Degree	Rank	Time	Credentials State Lic.	NCC	Email
Buchholz	Carol	B	PhD	Assistant Professor	>81		Y	Carol.E. Buchholz@ndsu.edu
Hall	Brenda	S	EdD	Associate Professor	>81		Y	brenda.hall@ndsu.edu
Nelson	Jill	R	PhD	Assistant Professor	>81		Y	Jill.R.Nelson@ndsu.edu
Nielsen	Robert	C	EdD	Full Professor	>81	Y	N	Robert.Nielsen@ndsu.edu

Percent of faculty with NCC certification: 75%

Other Certifications Held By Faculty Members: Certified School Counselor, LPC, LPC Supervisor

Enrollment and Admission Requirements

Degree	Program	Gender F	M	Yearly Admit	Grad	GRE Total	MAT	Master	GPA	Work Exp	Letters	Interview
MEd	Community Counseling	18	2	12	10	0		Y	3		3	Y
MEd	School Counseling	36	3	12	11	0			3		3	Y
PhD	Counselor Education	12	4	4	2	0		Y	3		3	Y

Graduation Requirements

Degree	Program	Academic Hours Sem	Qtr	Clock Hours Pract	Intern	Thesis	Examinations Comp	CPCE	Oral	Portfolio
MEd	Community Counseling	54		100	900		Y	Y		N
MEd	School Counseling	48		100	900		Y	Y		N
PhD	Counselor Education	71		100	600	Y	Y	N	Y	N

NH: Antioch University New England

40 Avon Street
Keene, NH 03431
United States of America
www.antiochne.edu

Dean
Carlotta J. Willis, Program Director, CMHC
40 Avon Street
Keene, NH 03431
United States of America

Administrator
Cynthia Feiker, Administrative Assistant
United States of America
(603) 357-3122; fax: NP
cwillis@antioch.edu

CSI Chapter, Name   N
Regionally Accredited   Y
Financial Aid   Y

Satellite Campus: N
International Students: Y
Number of International Students: 3-5 in related program (DMT)

Program Uniqueness

Dance movement therapy and counseling program. One day a week model for Clinical Mental Health Counseling program.

Faculty Research
NP

% faculty in professional counseling practice: NP

Program Accreditation

CACREP: Mental Health Counseling

Degree Programs
NP

Distance learning: N; % courses on-line: NP

Other Counseling Related Programs
NP

Faculty and Student Ethnicity
NP

Faculty
NP

Percent of faculty with NCC certification: NP

Other Credentials Held By Faculty Members
NP

Enrollment and Admission Requirements
NP

Graduation Requirements
NP

NH: Plymouth State University

17 High Street MSC 11
Plymouth, NH 03264
United States of America
http://www.plymouth.edu/graduate/counseling/index.html

Dean
George Tuthill
Interim Associate Vice-President for Graduate Studies
17 High Street MSC 11
Plymouth, NH 03264
United States of America

Administrator
Gail Mears
Department of Counselor Education and School Psychology
17 High Street, MSC 11
Plymouth, NH 03264
United States of America
(603) 535-2485; fax: (603) 535-2572
gmears@plymouth.edu

CSI Chapter, Name N
Regionally Accredited Y
Financial Aid Y

Satellite Campus: N
International Students: Y
Number of International Students: 5

Program Uniqueness

The counselor education program at Plymouth State University has several unique aspects. In addition to master's degree programs in school and mental health counseling, the department offers self-designed master's programs with foci in conflict in families, eating disorders and parenting education. Post-master's degree programs (Certificate of Advanced Graduate Studies) are available in school and mental health counseling and play therapy.

Faculty Research

Gary Goodnough: school counseling national standards, group counseling in schools, principals' perspectives on school counseling and integral school counseling. Gail Mears: cognitive complexity and relational aspects of supervision. Leo Sandy: service learning, peace education and faculty development. Hridaya Hall: meditation and breath therapy. Michael Fischler: multiculturalism and diversity issues.

33% faculty in professional counseling practice.

Program Accreditation

CACREP: Mental Health Counseling; **CACREP:** School Counseling

Degree Programs

Degree	Program	Contact
MEd	Mental Health Counseling	Dr. Gail Mears
M	School Counseling	Dr. Gary Goodnough
Advanced Graduate Certificate	Mental Health Counseling	Dr. Gail F. Mears
Advanced Graduate Certificate	School Counseling	Dr. Gary Goodnough

Distance learning: Y; 30% courses on-line

Other Counseling Related Programs
NP

Faculty and Student Ethnicity

Faculty	**Master's**	**Specialist**	**Doctoral**
Caucasian	African-American	African-American	
	Asian-American	Caucasian	
	Caucasian		
	Latino/Latina		

Faculty

Name			Highest Degree	Rank	Time	Credentials State Lic.	NCC	Email
Fischler	Michael	L	EdD	Full Professor	<21	N	N	mfischle@plymouth.edu
Goodnough	Gary	E	PhD	Full Professor	>81	Y	Y	ggoodno@plymouth.edu
Hall	K.	H	PhD	Assistant Professor		Y	Y	kehall@plymouth.edu
McNally	Heather		PhD	Adjunct		Y	N	hemcnally@plymouth.edu
Mears	Gail	F	PsyD	Chair	>81	Y	N	gmears@plymouth.edu
Sandy	Leo	R	EdD	Full Professor	<21	N	N	lsandy@plymouth.edu
Whelley	Peter	T	MS	Adjunct	<21	N	N	pwhelley@plymouth.edu

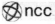 nbcc.   Percent of faculty with NCC certification: 33%   ncc

Other Credentials Held By Faculty Members
NP

Enrollment and Admission Requirements

Degree	Program	Gender F	Gender M	Yearly Admit	Yearly Grad	GRE Total	MAT	Master	GPA	Work Exp	Letters	Interview
MEd	Mental Health Counseling	4	4	15	8	0	50	Y	3		3	Y
M	School Counseling	25	5	15	8	0	50	Y	3		3	Y
AGC	Mental Health Counseling			5	2			Y			3	Y
AGC	School Counseling			5	2						3	Y

Graduation Requirements

Degree	Program	Academic Hours Sem	Qtr	Clock Hours Pract	Intern	Thesis	Examinations Comp	CPCE	Oral	Portfolio
MEd	Mental Health Counseling	63		100	900	N	N	N	N	N
M	School Counseling	48		100	600	N	N	N	N	Y
AGC	Mental Health Counseling	33				N				
AGC	School Counseling	33				Y				

NJ: Monmouth University

Department of Educational Leadership, School Counseling and Special Education
400 Cedar Ave.
West Long Branch, NJ 07764
United States of America
http://www.monmouth.edu/academics/schools/education/student_information/Gra
dPrograms.asp#Counseling

Dean

Lynn Romeo, Dean of the School of Education
School of Education
400 Cedar Ave.
West Long Branch, NJ 07764
United States of America

Administrator

Tina R. Paone, Assistant Professor
400 Cedar Ave.
West Long Branch, NJ 07764
United States of America
(732) 263-5291; fax: (732) 263-5710
tpaone@monmouth.edu

CSI Chapter, Name   NP
Regionally Accredited Y
Financial Aid   Y

Satellite Campus: N
International Students: N
Number of International students: 0

Program Uniqueness
NP

Faculty Research
NP

% faculty in professional counseling practice: NP

Program Accreditation

CACREP: Mental Health Counseling; **CACREP:** School Counseling

Degree Programs
NP

Distance learning: N; 25% courses on-line

Other Counseling Related Programs
NP

Faculty and Student Ethnicity
NP

Faculty
NP

Percent of faculty with NCC certification: NP

Other Credentials Held By Faculty Members
NP

Enrollment and Admission Requirements
NP

Graduation Requirements
NP

NJ: Montclair State University

Department of Counseling & Educational Leadership
UN 3162 1 Normal Avenue
Montclair, NJ 07043
United States of America

Dean   NP

Administrator   NP

CSI Chapter, Name   NP
Regionally Accredited NP
Financial Aid   NP

Satellite Campus: NP
International Students: NP
Number of International Students: NP

Program Uniqueness
NP

Faculty Research
NP

% faculty in professional counseling practice: NP

Program Accreditation

CACREP: Community Counseling; **CACREP:** School Counseling; **CACREP:** Student Affairs

Degree Programs
NP

Distance learning: NP; % courses on-line: NP

Other Counseling Related Programs
NP

Faculty and Student Ethnicity
NP

Faculty
NP

Percent of faculty with NCC certification: NP

Other Credentials Held By Faculty Members
NP

Enrollment and Admission Requirements
NP

Graduation Requirements
NP

NJ: Rowan University

201 Mullica Hill Road
Glassboro, NJ 08028
United States of America

Dean   NP

Administrator   NP

CSI Chapter, Name   NP
Regionally Accredited NP
Financial Aid   NP

Satellite Campus: NP
International Students: NP
Number of International Students: NP

Program Uniqueness
NP

Faculty Research
NP

% faculty in professional counseling practice: NP

Degree Programs
NP

Distance learning: NP; % courses on-line: NP

Other Counseling Related Programs
NP

Faculty and Student Ethnicity
NP

Faculty
NP

Percent of faculty with NCC certification: NP

Other Credentials Held By Faculty Members
NP

Enrollment and Admission Requirements
NP

Graduation Requirements
NP

NJ: William Paterson University

300 Pompton Rd.
Wayne, NJ 07470
United States of America
www.wpunj.edu/coe

Dean   Candice Burns
                      College of Education

Administrator   Paula Danzinger, Director
                      Professional Counseling Program
                      1600 Valley Road
                      Wayne, NJ 07470
                      United States of America
                      (973) 720-3085; fax: NP
                      danzingerp@wpunj.edu

CSI Chapter, Name   Y, Alpha Beta Chi
Regionally Accredited Y
Financial Aid   Y

Satellite Campus: N
International Students: NP
Number of International Students: NP

Program Uniqueness
NP

Faculty Research

Faculty research interests include suicide in adolescents, crisis intervention, violence in the
schools, grandparents raising grandchildren with AIDS, ethical implications of managed mental
health care, counselor licensure issues and ageism in mental health professionals.

33% faculty in professional counseling practice.

Program Accreditation

CACREP: Clinical Metal Health Counseling; **CACREP:** School Counseling

Degree Programs

Degree	*Program*	*Contact*
MEd	Mental Health Counseling	Paula R. Danzinger, Ph.D.
MEd	School Counseling	Paula R. Danzinger, Ph.D.

Distance learning: N; 1% courses on-line

Other Counseling Related Programs

Psychology

Faculty and Student Ethnicity

Faculty	**Master's**	**Specialist**	**Doctoral**
Asian	African-American		
Caucasian	Asian-American		
	Caucasian		
	Latino/Latina		

Faculty

Name			Highest Degree	Rank	Time	Credentials State Lic.	NCC	Email
Catarina	Mathilda		PhD	Associate Professor	>81	Y	N	catarinam@wpunj.ed
Danzinger	Paula	R	PhD	Associate Professor and Director of Counselor Education		Y	Y	danzingerp@wpunj.edu
Decker	Karen			Instructor		Y	Y	deckerk1@wpunj.edu
Heluk, Jr.	Henry		PhD	Assistant Professor	>81	Y	N	helukh@wpunj.edu
VanderGast	Timothy		PhD	Assistant Professor		Y	Y	vandergastt@wpunj.edu

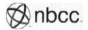 Percent of faculty with NCC certification: 60%

Other Credentials Held By Faculty Members: ACS, Approved Clinical Supervisor, CCMHC, Certified School Counselor, CSC, LPC

Enrollment and Admission Requirements

Degree	Program	Gender F M	Yearly Admit Grad	Total	GRE	MAT	Master	GPA	Work Exp	Letters	Interview
MEd	Mental Health Counseling	10	15 10	0	400	Y		2.75		2	Y
MEd	School Counseling		40 35	0	400	Y		2.75		2	Y

Graduation Requirements

Degree	Program	Academic Hours Sem Qtr	Clock Hours Pract	Intern	Thesis	Examinations Comp	CPCE	Oral	Portfolio
MEd	Mental Health Counseling	60	100	600	N	N	Y		Y
MEd	School Counseling	48	100	600	N		Y		Y

NV: University of Nevada

Department of Counseling and Educational Psychology/281
Reno, NV 89557-0213
United States of America
http://www.unr.edu/educ/cep/cepindex.html

Dean

William Sparkman
College of Education
Reno, NV 89557
United States of America

Administrator

Thomas Harrison, Professor and Chair
Department of Educational Psychology, Counseling,
and Human Development/281
Reno, NV 89557-0213
United States of America
(775) 682-7318; fax: (775) 784-1990
tch@unr.edu

CSI Chapter, Name   NP
Regionally Accredited Y
Financial Aid   Y

Satellite Campus: N
International Students: Y
Number of International Students: 3

Program Uniqueness

The Educational Psychology, Counseling, and Human Development Department includes the counseling program, the educational psychology program and the human development and family studies program. The department includes nationally recognized faculty scholars in counseling, educational psychology, information technology, child and family studies, and research and statistics. Faculty members are prolific researchers and publishers. Faculty members are also excellent teachers. Doctoral students collaborate with faculty in terms of research, publications, teaching and service activities. Master's students are also engaged in research activities.

Faculty Research

NP

40% faculty in professional counseling practice.

Program Accreditation

CACREP: College Counseling; **CACREP:** Community Counseling; **CACREP:** Counselor Education and Supervision; **CACREP:** Marital, Couple and Family Counseling/Therapy; **CACREP:** School Counseling

Degree Programs

Degree	*Program*	*Contact*
M	Addictions Counseling	Thomas Harrison
M	Community Counseling	Thomas Harrison
M	School Counseling	Jill Packman
M	Student Affairs	Mary Maples
S	Community Counseling	Thomas Harrison
S	School Counseling	Jill Packman
S	Student Affairs	Mary Maples
EdD	Addictions Counseling	Thomas Harrison
PhD	Addictions Counseling	Thomas Harrison
EdD	Community Counseling	Thomas Harrison
PhD	Community Counseling	Thomas Harrison

EdD	Counselor Education	Marlowe Smaby
PhD	Counselor Education	Marlowe Smaby
EdD	School Counseling	Marlowe Smaby
PhD	School Counseling	Marlowe Smaby
EdD	Student Affairs	Mary Maples
PhD	Student Affairs	Mary Maples

Distance learning: Y; 20% courses on-line

Other Counseling Related Programs

Clinical Social Workers
Communications
International Studies
Psychiatric Nurses
Psychiatrists
Psychology

Faculty and Student Ethnicity

Faculty	**Master's**	**Specialist**	**Doctoral**
Asian	African-American	African-American	African-American
Caucasian	Asian-American	Asian-American	Caucasian
Latino/Latina	Caucasian	Caucasian	Latino/Latina
	Latino/Latina	Latino/Latina	Native American
	Multiracial	Multiracial	
	Native American	Native American	

Faculty

Name		Highest Degree	Rank	Time	Credentials State Lic.	NCC	Email
Abney	Paul	PhD	Assistant Professor	>81		Y	abney@unr.edu
D'Andrea	Livia	PhD	Associate Professor	61-80		N	livia@unr.edu
Harrison	Thomas	PhD	Associate Professor	>81		N	tch@unr.edu
Maples	Mary	PhD	Full Professor	>81		Y	maples@unr.edu
Packman	Jill	PhD	Assistant Professor	>81		Y	packman@unr.edu
Smaby	Marlowe	PhD	Full Professor	>81		Y	smaby@unr.edu
Torres-Rivera	Edil	PhD	Associate Professor	>81		Y	torre_e@unr.edu

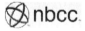 Percent of faculty with NCC certification: 71%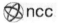

Other Credentials Held By Faculty Members
NP

Enrollment and Admission Requirements

Degree	Program	Gender F	Gender M	Yearly Admit	Yearly Grad	GRE Total	MAT	Master	GPA	Work Exp	Letters	Interview
M	Addictions Counseling	8	2	5	3	750			3	2	3	
M	Community Counseling	35	20	15	12	750			3	2	3	
M	School Counseling	35	20	15	12	750			3	2	3	
M	Student Affairs	8	2	5	3	750			3	2	3	
S	Community Counseling	35	20	15	12					2	3	
S	School Counseling	35	20	15	12					2	3	
S	Student Affairs	8	2	5	3					2	3	
EdD	Addictions Counseling	4	1	1	1	1000		Y	4	2	3	Y
PhD	Addictions Counseling	4	1	1	1	1000		Y	4	2	3	Y
EdD	Community Counseling	4	1	2	1	1000		Y	4	2	3	Y
PhD	Community Counseling	4	1	2	1	1000		Y	4	2	3	Y
EdD	Counselor Education											
PhD	Counselor Education											
EdD	School Counseling			2	1	1000		Y	4	2	3	Y
PhD	School Counseling			2	1	1000		Y	4	2	3	Y
EdD	Student Affairs			1	1	1000		Y	4	2	3	Y
PhD	Student Affairs			1	1	1000		Y	4	2	3	Y

Graduation Requirements

Degree	Program	Academic Hours		Clock Hours		Examinations				
		Sem	Qtr	Pract	Intern	Thesis	Comp	CPCE	Oral	Portfolio
M	Addictions Counseling	60		100	600		Y	Y		
M	Community Counseling	60		100	600		Y	Y		
M	School Counseling	60		100	600		Y	Y		
M	Student Affairs	60		100	600			Y		
S	Community Counseling	35			600	Y	Y	Y		
S	School Counseling	35			600	Y	Y	Y		
S	Student Affairs	35			600	Y	Y	Y		
EdD	Addictions Counseling	100			600	Y	Y	Y	Y	
PhD	Addictions Counseling	100			600	Y	Y	Y	Y	
EdD	Community Counseling	100			600	Y	Y	Y	Y	
PhD	Community Counseling	100			600	Y	Y	Y	Y	
EdD	Counselor Education	100			600	Y	Y	Y	Y	
PhD	Counselor Education	100			600	Y	Y	Y		Y
EdD	School Counseling	100			600	Y	Y			Y
PhD	School Counseling	100			600	Y	Y			Y
EdD	Student Affairs	100			600	Y	Y	Y	Y	
PhD	Student Affairs	100			600	Y	Y	Y	Y	

NV: University of Nevada, Las Vegas

4505 Maryland Parkway
Las Vegas, NV 89154-3001
United States of America
http://education.unlv.edu/ced/

Dean
William Speer, Professor and Interim Dean
4505 Maryland Parkway
College of Education
Las Vegas, NV 89154-3001
United States of America

Administrator
Dale-Elizabeth Pehrsson, Professor and Chair
4505 Maryland Parkway
Las Vegas, NV 89154-3001
United States of America
(702) 895-5994; fax: NP
dale.pehrsson@unlv.edu

CSI Chapter, Name NP
Regionally Accredited Y
Financial Aid Y

Satellite Campus: N
International Students: Y
Number of International Students: 2

Program Uniqueness

UNLV is located in a dynamic international city that provides students with rich cultural learning and diverse experiences. UNLV's Counselor Education program offers extensive training in professional school counseling, clinical mental health counseling and addictions counseling. Further, our underpinning focus is an ethic of social caring and justice. We offer a con-joint Ph.D. in Counselor Education and Educational Psychology, and our students gain excellent research skills in addition to becoming professional counselor educators and supervisors.

Faculty Research
NP

0% faculty in professional counseling practice.

Program Accreditation

CACREP: Mental Health Counseling; **CACREP:** School Counseling

Degree Programs

Degree	Program	Contact
MS	Clinical Mental Health Counseling	
MEd	School Counseling	
	Counselor Education and Supervision	

Distance learning: Y; 33% courses on-line

Other Counseling Related Programs
NP

Faculty and Student Ethnicity
NP

Faculty
NP

Percent of faculty with NCC certification: NP

Other Credentials Held By Faculty Members
NP

Enrollment and Admission Requirements

Degree	Program	Gender F	M	Yearly Admit	Grad	GRE Total	MAT	Master	GPA	Work Exp	Letters	Interview
MS	Clinical Mental Health Counseling	17	8	25	20			Y				Y
MEd	School Counseling	22	3	25	20			Y				Y
	Counselor Education and Supervision	5	1	6	2							

Graduation Requirements

Degree	Program	Academic Hours Sem	Qtr	Clock Hours Pract	Intern	Thesis	Comp	CPCE	Oral	Portfolio
MS	Clinical Mental Health Counseling	60		100	900	N	Y	N	N	Y
MEd	School Counseling	48		100	600	N	Y	N	N	Y
	Counselor Education and Supervision									

NY: Canisius College

2001 Main Street
Buffalo, NY 14208-1098
United States of America
www.canisius.edu

Dean Shawn O'Rourke, Associate Dean of Graduate Education
School of Education and Human Services
Canisius College
2001 Main Street
Buffalo, NY 14208
United States of America

Administrator E. Christine Moll, Department Chairperson
2001 Main Street
Buffalo, NY 14208-1098
United States of America
(716) 888-3287; fax: (716) 888-3299
moll@canisius.edu

CSI Chapter, Name Y, Psi Chi Gamma
Regionally Accredited Y
Financial Aid N

Satellite Campus: N
International Students: Y
Number of International Students: 5

Program Uniqueness

Programs in community mental health and school counseling prepare students for a NYS License in Mental Health Counseling or NYS Certification in school counseling in a student-friendly atmosphere. Specialty work toward substance abuse (CASAC) and rehabilitation counseling (CRC) certification is available. Our location within the city of Buffalo is close to an international border. Our commitment to diversity makes Canisius a great choice for international students. The Graduate Division at Canisius College is one of the most respected schools in Western New York.

Faculty Research

Interests include, but are not limited to, adult development and aging, bereavement, ethics, learned optimism, school violence and school safety, supervision of counselors, and wellness.

60% faculty in professional counseling practice.

Program Accreditation

CACREP: Community Counseling; **CACREP:** School Counseling

Degree Programs

Degree	*Program*	*Contact*
MS	Community-Mental Health Counseling	E. Christine Moll
MS	School Counseling	E. Christine Moll

Distance learning: N; 5% courses on-line

Other Counseling Related Programs
NP

Faculty and Student Ethnicity

Faculty	**Master's**	**Specialist**	**Doctoral**
Asian-American	African-American		
Caucasian	Caucasian		
	Latino/Latina		
	Native American		

Faculty

Name			Highest Degree	Rank	Time	Credentials State Lic.	NCC	Email
Farrugia	David		EdD	Full Professor	>81	Y	Y	Farriguia@canisius.edu
Fetter	Holly	T	PhD	Associate Professor	>81	N	Y	tanigosh@canisius.edu
Lenhardt	Ann Marie		PhD	Full Professor	>81	Y	Y	lenharda@canisius.edu
Moll	B. Christine		PhD	Associate Professor and Chair	>81	Y	Y	moll@canisius.edu
Rutter	Michael		EdD	Associate Professor	>81		Y	rutter@canisius.edu

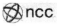 Percent of faculty with NCC certification: 100%

Other Credentials Held By Faculty Members: Licensed Psychologist, LMHC, LMHP

Enrollment and Admission Requirements

Degree	Program	Gender F	M	Yearly Admit	Grad	GRE Total	MAT	Master	GPA	Work Exp	Letters	Interview
MS	Community-Mental Health Counseling	50	20	35	35	0		Y	2.7		2	Y
MS	School Counseling	50	20	35	35	0		Y	2.7		2	Y

Graduation Requirements

Degree	Program	Academic Hours Sem	Qtr	Clock Hours Pract	Intern	Examinations Thesis	Comp	CPCE	Oral	Portfolio
MS	Community-Mental Health Counseling	60		100	600	N	Y	Y	N	N
MS	School Counseling	48		100	600	N	Y	Y	N	N

NY: St. John Fisher College

3690 East Avenue
Rochester, NY 14618
United States of America
www.sjfc.edu

Dean   Dianne Cooney-Miner, Dean
Wegman`s School of Nursing
3690 East Avenue
Rochester, NY 14618
United States of America

Administrator   Signe M. Kastberg, Ph.D., NCC, LMHC, Program Director
3690 East Avenue
Rochester, NY 14618
United States of America
(585) 385-7222; fax: (585) 385-7276
skastberg@sjfc.edu

CSI Chapter, Name   N
Regionally Accredited Y
Financial Aid   Y

Satellite Campus: N
International Students: Y
Number of International Students: NP

Program Uniqueness
NP

Faculty Research
NP

75% faculty in professional counseling practice.

Program Accreditation

CACREP: Mental Health Counseling

Degree Programs
NP

Distance learning: N; 0% courses on-line

Other Counseling Related Programs
NP

Faculty and Student Ethnicity
NP

Faculty
NP

Percent of faculty with NCC certification: NP

Other Credentials Held By Faculty Members
NP

Enrollment and Admission Requirements
NP

Graduation Requirements
NP

NY: St. Lawrence University

Atwood Hall
Canton, NY 13617
United States of America
www.stlawu.edu/education

Dean   Arthur J. Clark, Professor, Coordinator
Counseling and Human Development Program
Atwood Hall
Canton, NY 13617
United States of America

Administrator   NP

CSI Chapter, Name   N
Regionally Accredited Y
Financial Aid   Y

Satellite Campus: N
International Students: Y
Number of International Students: 2

Program Uniqueness
NP

Faculty Research
NP

20% faculty in professional counseling practice.

Degree Programs

Degree	*Program*	*Contact*
MS	Mental Health Counseling	

Distance learning: N; 0% courses on-line

Other Counseling Related Programs
NP

Faculty and Student Ethnicity
NP

Faculty
NP

Percent of faculty with NCC certification: NP

Other Credentials Held By Faculty Members
NP

Enrollment and Admission Requirements

Degree	Program	Gender		Yearly		GRE	MAT	Master	GPA	Work	Letters	Interview
		F	M	Admit	Grad	Total				Exp		
MS	Mental Health Counseling	6	2	6	4							

Graduation Requirements

Degree	Program	Academic Hours		Clock Hours			Examinations				
		Sem	Qtr	Pract	Intern	Thesis	Comp	CPCE	Oral	Portfolio
MS	Mental Health Counseling									

OH: Kent State University

Counseling and Human Development Services
310 White Hall
P.O. Box 5190
Kent, OH 44242-0001
United States of America
http://www.kent.edu/ehhs/chds/index.cfm

Dean
Dan Mahony
402 White Hall
P.O. Box 5190
Kent State University
Kent, OH 44242-0001
United States of America

Administrator
Mary Dellmann-Jenkins,School Director
405 White Hall
P.O. Box 5190
Kent State University
Kent, OH 44242-0001
United States of America
(330) 672-6958; fax: NP

CSI Chapter, Name   Y, Kappa Sigma Upsilon
Regionally Accredited Y
Financial Aid   Y

Satellite Campus: N
International Students: Y
Number of International Students: 5

Program Uniqueness

The program has an active on-site counseling center in which many students complete their practica experience.

Faculty Research

Research interests include group work, supervision of counseling, crisis intervention, school counselor preparation, multicultural counseling skill training, CACREP standards, substance abuse, family counseling, and integration of technology in counseling and counselor education.

% faculty in professional counseling practice: NP

Program Accreditation

CACREP: Community Counseling; **CACREP:** Counselor Education and Supervision; **CACREP:** School Counseling

Degree Programs

Degree	Program	Contact
M	Clinical Mental Health Counseling	Dr. Jason McGlothlin
M	School Counseling	Dr. Jason McGlothlin
EdS	Counseling	Dr. McGlothlin or Dr. West
PhD	Counseling and Human Development Services	Dr. John West

Distance learning: N; 5% courses on-line

Other Counseling Related Programs
NP

Faculty and Student Ethnicity

Faculty	**Master's**	**Specialist**	**Doctoral**
Caucasian	African-American	African-American	African-American
	Asian-American	Asian-American	Asian
	Caucasian	Caucasian	Caucasian
	Latino/Latina	Latino/Latina	Latino/Latina
	Multiracial	Multiracial	Multiracial

Faculty

Name			Highest Degree	Rank	Time	State Lic.	NCC	Email
Bubenzer	Donald		PhD	Professor Emeritus	<21	Y	N	dbubenze@kent.edu
Cox	Jane		PhD	Associate Professor	>81	Y	N	jcox8@kent.edu
Unilita	Philip		PhD	Assistant Professor	>81	N	Y	
Guillot-Miller	Lynne		PhD	Associate Professor	>81	N	N	lguillot@kent.edu
Jencius	Marty		PhD	Associate Professor	>81	N	N	mjencius@kent.edu
McGlothlin	Jason	M	PhD	Associate Professor	>81	Y	N	jmcgloth@kent.edu
Miller	Jason	L	PhD	Director of the Counseling and Human Development Center	<21	Y	N	jmille4@kent.edu
Osborn	Cynthia	J	PhD	Full Professor	>81	Y	N	cosborn@kent.edu
Page	Betsy	J	EdD	Associate Professor		Y	Y	bpage@kent.edu
Rainey	John	S	PhD	Assistant Professor	>81	N	N	jrainey@kent.edu
Savickas	Mark	L	PhD	Adjunct	<21	Y	N	msavakas@kent.edu
West	John	D	EdD	Full Professor		Y	N	jwest@kent.edu

   Percent of faculty with NCC certification: 17%

Other Credentials Held By Faculty Members: Approved Clinical Supervisor, CMFT

Enrollment and Admission Requirements

Degree	Program	Gender F	Gender M	Yearly Admit	Yearly Grad	GRE Total	MAT	Master	GPA	Work Exp	Letters	Interview
M	Clinical Mental Health Counseling	90	30	40	34	0		Y	2.75		2	Y
M	School Counseling	52	5	32	25	0		Y	2.75		2	Y
EdS	Counseling	9	1	4	2	0		Y	3		2	Y
PhD	Counseling and Human Development Services	45	15	14	10			Y	3.5		2	Y

Graduation Requirements

Degree	Program	Academic Hours Sem	Qtr	Clock Hours Pract	Clock Hours Intern	Thesis	Comp	CPCE	Oral	Portfolio
M	Clinical Mental Health Counseling	60		100	600	N	Y	N	N	N
M	School Counseling	49		100	600	N	Y	N	N	N
EdS	Counseling	30		100	600	N	N	N	N	N
PhD	Counseling and Human Development Services	104		100	600	Y	Y	N	Y	N

OH: Ohio University

201 McCracken Hall
Athens, OH 45701-2979
United States of America
http://www.ohiou.edu/education/index.html

Dean

Renee Middleton
133 McCracken Hall
Ohio University
Athens, OH 45778
United States of America

Administrator

Thomas Davis, Ph.D., PCC, Professor
370 McCracken Hall
Athens, OH 45701-2979
United States of America
(740) 593-4442; fax: NP

CSI Chapter, Name   Y
Regionally Accredited Y
Financial Aid   Y

Satellite Campus: NP
International Students: Y
Number of International Students: 10%

Program Uniqueness

Close faculty-student interaction. Aid in the design of one's program to fit own personal goal.

Faculty Research
NP

% faculty in professional counseling practice: NP

Program Accreditation

CACREP: Clinical Mental Health Counseling; **CACREP:** Counselor Education and Supervision; **CACREP:** School Counseling; **CORE:** Rehabilitation Counseling

Degree Programs

Degree	Program	Contact
M	Community Counseling	Pat Beamish
M	Rehabilitation Counseling	Jerry Olsheski
M	School Counseling	Tracy Leinbaugh
PhD	Counselor Education	Tom Davis

Distance learning: NP; % courses on-line: NP

Other Counseling Related Programs
NP

Faculty and Student Ethnicity

Faculty	Master's	Specialist	Doctoral
African-American	African-American		African-American
Caucasian	Asian-American		Asian
Multiracial	Caucasian		Caucasian
	Latino/Latina		Latino/Latina
	Multiracial		Multiracial
	Native American		Native American

Faculty

Name		Highest Degree	Rank	Time	Credentials State Lic.	NCC	Email
Beamish	Patricia	EdD	Associate Professor	>81	Y	N	beamish@ohio.edu
Davis	Thomas	PhD	Full Professor	>81	Y	N	davist@ohio.edu
Doston	Glenn	PhD	Full Professor	>81		N	doston@ohio.edu
Hazler	Richard	EdD	Full Professor	>81	Y	Y	hazler@ohio.edu
Leinbaugh	Tracy	PhD	Assistant Professor	>81	Y	Y	leinbaug@ohio.edu
Levitt	Dana	PhD	Assistant Professor	>81		N	levitt@ohio.edu
Olsheski	Jerry	PhD	Associate Professor	>81	Y	N	olsheski@ohio.edu
Stump	Earl	PhD	Instructor		Y	N	Stump@ohio.edu
Sweeney	Thomas	PhD	Adjunct	22-40		N	

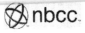 **nbcc.**   Percent of faculty with NCC certification: 22%   **ncc**

Other Credentials Held By Faculty Members
NP

Enrollment and Admission Requirements

Degree	Program	Gender F	M	Yearly Admit	Grad	GRE Total	MAT	Master	GPA	Work Exp	Letters	Interview
M	Community Counseling	20	10	30	25	900			3		3	
M	Rehabilitation Counseling			7	7	0			3		3	
M	School Counseling			8	8	900			3		3	
PhD	Counselor Education			12	12	1000		Y			3	Y

Graduation Requirements

Degree	Program	Academic Hours Sem	Qtr	Clock Hours Pract	Intern	Examinations Thesis	Comp	CPCE	Oral	Portfolio
M	Community Counseling					N	N	N	N	Y
M	Rehabilitation Counseling									
M	School Counseling									
PhD	Counselor Education				720	Y	Y			

OH: University of Cincinnati

Teachers College Building 526 M. L. 0068
Cincinnati, OH 45221-0068
United States of America
www.uc.edu/counselingprogram

Dean

Professor Lawrence J. Johnson
College of Education, Criminal Justice and Human Services
Cincinnati, OH 45221-0002
United States of America

Administrator

Mei Tang, Professor and Program Director
Dyer Hall 429
M. L. 0068
University of Cincinnati
Cincinnati, OH 45221-0068
United States of America
(513) 556-3335; fax: (513) 556-3898
mei.tang@uc.edu

CSI Chapter, Name   Y, Upsilon Chi Chi
Regionally Accredited Y
Financial Aid   Y

Satellite Campus: N
International Students: Y
Number of International Students: 2

Program Uniqueness

Our accredited programs in school counseling, mental health counseling, and counselor education and supervision (doctoral) emphasize an ecological orientation with a focus on diversity and underserved populations.

Faculty Research

Ecological counseling, supervision, problem-based learning, mental health services to the underserved, career development, group work, prevention, students with disabilities, substance abuse prevention and treatment, conflict resolution, diversity and social justice.

30% faculty in professional counseling practice.

Program Accreditation

CACREP: Counselor Education and Supervision; **CACREP:** Mental Health Counseling; **CACREP:** School Counseling

CACREP

Degree Programs

Degree	Program	Contact
MA	Mental Health Counseling	F. Robert Wilson, Ph.D.
MEd	School Counseling	Kerry Sebera, Ph. D.
EdD	Counselor Education and Supervision	Ellen Cook

Distance learning: N; 10% courses on-line

Other Counseling Related Programs

Clinical Social Workers
Communications
Psychiatric Nurses
Psychiatrists
Psychology

Faculty and Student Ethnicity

Faculty	Master's	Specialist	Doctoral
African-American	African-American		African-American
Asian	Caucasian		Asian
Caucasian	Multiracial		Caucasian
			Latino/Latina
			Multiracial
			Native American

Faculty

Name			Highest Degree	Rank	Time	Credentials State Lic.	NCC	Email
Brubaker	Michael	D.	PhD	Assistant Professor			Y	michael.brubaker@uc.edu
Conyne	Robert	K.	PhD	Professor Emeritus		Y	N	robert.conyne@uc.edu
Cook	Ellen	P	PhD	Full Professor		Y	N	ellen.cook@uc.edu
Rothman	Jay		PhD	Visiting Professor	22-40		N	jay.rothman@uc.edu
Sebera	Kerry	E.	PhD	Assistant Professor		Y	N	kerry.sebera@uc.edu
Tang	Mei		PhD	Full Professor and Director of Graduate Program	>81	Y	N	mei.tang@uc.edu
Watson	Albert	L	PhD	Associate Professor		Y	N	albert.l.watson@uc.edu
Wilson	Frederick	R	PhD	Full Professor		Y	Y	wilsonfr@ucmail.uc.edu
Yager	Geoffrey	G	PhD	Full Professor		Y	Y	geof.yager@uc.edu

 nbcc.   Percent of faculty with NCC certification: 33%   ⊗ncc.

Other Credentials Held By Faculty Members: ACS, Approved Clinical Supervisor, PCC

Enrollment and Admission Requirements

Degree	Program	Gender F	Gender M	Yearly Admit	Yearly Grad	GRE Total	MAT	Master	GPA	Work Exp	Letters	Interview
MA	Mental Health Counseling	19	3	22	22	900		Y	3		3	Y
MEd	School Counseling	12	2	14	14	900		Y	3		3	Y
EdD	Counselor Education and Supervision	4	2	5	3	900		Y	3.25	0	3	Y

Graduation Requirements

Degree	Program	Academic Hours Sem	Academic Hours Qtr	Clock Hours Pract	Clock Hours Intern	Examinations Thesis	Comp	CPCE	Oral	Portfolio
MA	Mental Health Counseling		90	100	900	N	Y	Y	N	N
MEd	School Counseling		72	100	600	N	Y	Y	N	Y
EdD	Counselor Education and Supervision		90	100	600	Y	Y	N	Y	N

OH: Youngstown State University

1 University Plaza
Youngstown, OH 44555
United States of America
http://bcoe.ysu.coe

Dean	Dr. Phil Ginnetti

Dr. Phil Ginnetti
College of Education
1 University Plaza
Youngstown, OH 44555
United States of America

Administrator   Jake Protivnak, Counseling Program Coordinator
1 University Plaza
Youngstown, OH 44555
United States of America
(330) 941-3257; fax: (330) 941-2369
jjprotivnak@ysu.edu

CSI Chapter, Name   Y, Chi Sigma Iota
Regionally Accredited Y
Financial Aid   Y

Satellite Campus: N
International Students: Y
Number of International Students: 5

Program Uniqueness

Our program is focused on issues of poverty particularly related to urban populations. We have an active urban community clinic and a large number of assistantships.

Faculty Research

Character education, multicultural issues, domestic abuse, self-mutilation, school violence and bullying, female incarceration, cutting behavior, personality disorders, urban issues and poverty.

30% faculty in professional counseling practice.

Program Accreditation

CACREP: Community Counseling; **CACREP:** School Counseling; **CACREP:** Student Affairs

Degree Programs

Degree	*Program*	*Contact*
M	Community Counseling	Victoria White Kress
MS	School Counseling	Don Martin
M	Student Affairs	Deborah Jackson

Distance learning: N; 0% courses on-line

Other Counseling Related Programs
NP

Faculty and Student Ethnicity

Faculty	Master's	Specialist	Doctoral
	African-American		
	Asian-American		
	Caucasian		
	Latino/Latina		
	Multiracial		
	Native American		
	Pacific Islander		

Faculty

Name			Highest Degree	Rank	Time	Credentials State Lic.	NCC	Email
Jackson	Deborah		PhD	Assistant Professor	61-80		N	dljackson.01@ysu.edu
Kress	Victoria	W	PhD	Full Professor	61-80	Y	N	vewhite@ysu.edu
Martin	Don		PhD	Full Professor	61-80	Y	N	dmartin@ysu.edu
Miller	Kenneth		PhD	Full Professor	61-80	Y	Y	klmiller@ysu.edu
Paylo	Matt		PhD	Assistant Professor	22-40	Y	N	mpaylo@ysu.edu
Protivnak	Jake		PhD	Assistant Professor	61-80	Y	N	jprotivnak@yahoo.com

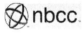 Percent of faculty with NCC certification: 17%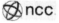

Other Credentials Held By Faculty Members: Licensed Psychologist, Licensed School Counselor, LPC, LPC Supervisor

Enrollment and Admission Requirements

Degree	Program	Gender F	M	Yearly Admit	Grad	GRE Total	MAT	Master	GPA	Work Exp	Letters	Interview
M	Community Counseling	70	30	40	20			Y	2.7		3	Y
MS	School Counseling			20	10			Y	2.8		2	Y
M	Student Affairs								2.7		3	Y

Graduation Requirements

Degree	Program	Academic Hours Sem	Qtr	Clock Hours Pract	Intern	Thesis	Comp	Examinations CPCE	Oral	Portfolio
M	Community Counseling	63		150	600	N	Y	Y	N	N
MS	School Counseling	52		150	600	N	Y	Y	N	N
M	Student Affairs	36		200	600	N	Y	N	N	N

OR: George Fox University

12753 SW 68th Avenue
Portland, OR 97223
United States of America
www.georgefox.edu/academics/graduate/counseling

Dean   Linda Samek, Dean of the School of Education

Administrator   Richard Shaw, D.MFT, Department Chair, Director
12753 SW 68th Avenue
Portland, OR 97223
United States of America
(503) 554-6142; fax: (503) 554-6111
jfreitag@georgefox.edu

CSI Chapter, Name   N
Regionally Accredited Y
Financial Aid   Y

Satellite Campus: Y
International Students: Y
Number of International Students: NP

Program Uniqueness

The members of the Graduate Department of Counseling faculty are active clinicians and educators with real life experience and training. The program has a purposeful integrative focus on the best of counselor education and Christ-based faith.

Faculty Research

Trauma (PTSD), play therapy, spirituality issues, supervision, and program distance writing.

70% faculty in professional counseling practice.

Degree Programs

Degree	*Program*	*Contact*
MA	Marriage and Family Counseling	Richard Shaw
MA	Mental Health Counseling	Richard Shaw
MA	School Counseling	Richard Shaw

Distance learning: N; % courses on-line: NP

Other Counseling Related Programs

Psychology

Faculty and Student Ethnicity

Faculty	**Master's**	**Specialist**	**Doctoral**
African-American	African-American		
Asian	Asian-American		
Caucasian	Caucasian		
Latino/Latina	Latino/Latina		
Multiracial	Multiracial		
Native American	Native American		
Other	Pacific Islander		

Faculty

Name		Highest Degree	Rank	Time	Credentials State Lic.	NCC	Email
Bearden	Steve	PhD	Assistant Professor	>81	N	N	
Berardi	Anna	PhD	Associate Professor	>81	Y	N	
Cox	Michelle	PhD	Assistant Professor	>81	Y	Y	
DeKruyf	Lorraine	PhD	Associate Professor	61-80	N	N	
Dempsey	Keith	PhD	Assistant Professor	>81	N	N	
Manock	David	PhD	Assistant Professor	>81	N	N	
Michael	Rand	DMin	Associate Professor	>81	Y	N	
Shaw	Richard	DMFT	Associate Professor and Director of Counselor Education	<21	Y	N	
Simpson	Bob	PhD	Assistant Professor	>81	N	N	
Sweeney	Daniel	PhD	Professor	>81	Y	N	

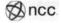 **nbcc**   Percent of faculty with NCC certification: 10%   **ncc**

Other Credentials Held By Faculty Members: AAMFT Approved Supervisor, AAMFT Clinical Member, Certified School Psychologist, LMFT, LMHC, MFCC, MFT

Enrollment and Admission Requirements

Degree	Program	Gender F	M	Yearly Admit	Grad	GRE Total	MAT	Master	GPA	Work Exp	Letters	Interview
MA	Marriage and Family Counseling	73	22	40	35	0		Y	3		3	Y
MA	Mental Health Counseling	99	24	40	35	0		Y	3		3	Y
MA	School Counseling		7	15	12	0		Y	3		3	Y

Graduation Requirements

Degree	Program	Academic Hours Sem	Qtr	Clock Hours Pract	Intern	Thesis	Comp	Examinations CPCE	Oral	Portfolio
MA	Marriage and Family Counseling	68		100	700	Y	Y			Y
MA	Mental Health Counseling	56		100	600	Y	Y			Y
MA	School Counseling	57		100	600	Y	Y			Y

OR: Oregon State University

Counseling Academic Unit
Department of Teacher and Counselor Education
College of Education
Oregon State University
4th floor, Waldo Hall
Corvallis, OR 97331-6403
United States of America
http://oregonstate.edu/education/programs/counseling.html

Dean

Sam Stern
College of Education
Oregon State University
4th floor, Waldo Hall
Corvallis, OR 97331-6403
United States of America

Administrator

Cass Dykeman, Lead
Counseling Academic Unit
Department of Teacher and Counselor Education
College of Education
Oregon State University
4th floor, Waldo Hall
Corvallis, OR 97331-8536
United States of America
(541) 737-8204; fax: (541) 737-2040
dykemanc@onid.orst.edu

CSI Chapter, Name   NP
Regionally Accredited Y
Financial Aid   Y

Satellite Campus: Y
International Students: N
Number of International Students: 0

Program Uniqueness

The faculty and students honor lived experiences of all individuals and affirm the concepts of D.R.I.V.E: Dignity, Respect, Integrity, Value, and Equality.

Faculty Research

School counseling, addictive counseling, career counseling, multicultural issues, play therapy, and group process.

20% faculty in professional counseling practice.

Program Accreditation

CACREP: Community Counseling; **CACREP:** Counselor Education and Supervision; **CACREP:** School Counseling

Degree Programs

Degree	*Program*	*Contact*
MS	Community Counseling	Gene Eakin
M	School Counseling	
PhD	Counselor Education	Cass Dykeman

Distance learning: N; 0% courses on-line

Other Counseling Related Programs

Have made transition of community counseling program to 90 quarter hour Clinical Mental Health Counselor program.

Faculty and Student Ethnicity

Faculty	**Master's**	**Specialist**	**Doctoral**
African-American	Asian-American		Caucasian
Caucasian	Caucasian		
Multiracial	Multiracial		
	Native American		

Faculty

Name			Highest Degree	Rank	Time	Credentials State Lic.	NCC	Email
Biles	Kathy		PhD	Instructor	>81		Y	
Blackman	Lorie		PhD	Instructor	41-60		N	lblackma@hotmail.com
Dykeman	Cass		PhD	Associate Professor	>81	N	Y	dykemanc@onid.orst.edu
Eakin	Gene	A	PhD	Instructor			N	gene.eakin@oregonstate.edu
McLain	Susan		MS	Instructor	41-60		N	
Mphande-Finn	Joyce	T	EdD	Instructor		Y	N	joyce.mphandefinn@osucascades.edu
Rubel	Deborah	J	PhD	Associate Professor	>81	Y	N	deborah.rubel@oregonstate.edu
Stauffer	Mark	D	PhD	Instructor	22-40	N	Y	mark@markstauffer.com
Strong	Teri		PhD	Instructor	22-40		N	strongt@oregonstate.edu
Stroud	Daniel		PhD	Instructor	>81		N	

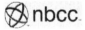 Percent of faculty with NCC certification: 30%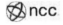

Other Credentials Held By Faculty Members: Approved Clinical Supervisor, Certified School Counselor, Certified School Psychologist, Licensed Psychologist, LPC, MAC, NCSC

Enrollment and Admission Requirements

Degree	Program	Gender F	M	Yearly Admit	Grad	GRE Total	MAT	Master	GPA	Work Exp	Letters	Interview
MS	Community Counseling	52	24	24	20	0		Y	3		3	Y
M	School Counseling	62	14	24	20	0		Y	3		3	Y
PhD	Counselor Education	35	9	14	10	0		Y	3		3	Y

Graduation Requirements

Degree	Program	Academic Hours Sem	Qtr	Clock Hours Pract	Intern	Thesis	Comp	Examinations CPCE	Oral	Portfolio
MS	Community Counseling		75	100	600				Y	Y
M	School Counseling		75	100	600				Y	Y
PhD	Counselor Education		150	100	600	Y	Y		Y	

OR: Portland State University

Graduate School of Education
P.O. Box 751
Portland, OR 97207
United States of America

Dean   Randy Hitz

Administrator   Rick Johnson, Ph.D., Department Chair
Counselor Education
Graduate School of Education
P.O. Box 751
Portland, OR 97207
United States of America
(503) 725-9764; fax: (503) 725-5599
johnsonp@pdx.edu

CSI Chapter, Name   NP
Regionally Accredited   Y
Financial Aid   Y

Satellite Campus: N
International Students: Y
Number of International Students: NP

Program Uniqueness

The Counselor Education Department offers specializations in school counseling; clinical mental health counseling; rehabilitation counseling; and marital, couples and family counseling. It is accredited by CACREP and CORE and in good standing with the licensure board. The in-house practicum clinic provides excellent supervision and receives referrals from schools and agencies from every sector of the city and surrounding areas. Internship placements abound, and classes are formatted for evenings and weekends. Faculty members are personable and bring diverse life experiences and teaching styles to our students.

Faculty Research

Psychosocial aspects of disability, youth at risk, grief and loss, suicide prevention, ethical decision-making, group work, theories of counseling and psychotherapy.

25% faculty in professional counseling practice.

Program Accreditation

CACREP: Community Counseling; **CACREP:** Marital, Couple and Family Counseling/Therapy; **CACREP:** School Counseling

Degree Programs

Degree	Program	Contact
M	Community Counseling	Russ Miars
M	Marriage and Family Counseling	Susan Halverson
M	Rehabilitation Counseling	Hancock Livneh
M	School Counseling	Lisa Aasheim

Distance learning: N; 0% courses on-line

Other Counseling Related Programs

Clinical Social Workers

Faculty and Student Ethnicity

Faculty	**Master's**	**Specialist**	**Doctoral**
African-American	African-American		
Asian	Asian-American		
Caucasian	Latino/Latina		
Native American	Multiracial		
	Native American		
	Pacific Islander		

Faculty

Name		Highest Degree	Rank	Time	Credentials State Lic.	NCC	Email
Aasheim	Lisa	PhD	Assistant Professor			Y	aasheim@pdx.edu
Anctil	Tina	PhD	Assistant Professor		Y	N	
Halverson	Susan	PhD	Assistant Professor	>81	Y	N	halversons@pdx.edu
Johnson	Rick	PhD	Associate Professor and Chair		Y	N	johnsonp@pdx.edu
Livneh	Hanoch	PhD	Full Professor	>81	Y	Y	livnehh@pdx.edu
Miars	Russ	PhD	Associate Professor	>81		N	miarsr@pdx.edu
Wosley-George	Liz	PhD	Associate Professor	>81	Y	N	wosleygeorgee@pdx.edu

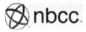 Percent of faculty with NCC certification: 29%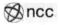

Other Credentials Held By Faculty Members: AAMFT Clinical Member, CRC, Licensed Psychologist, LPC

Enrollment and Admission Requirements

Degree	Program	Gender F M	Yearly Admit Grad	GRE Total	MAT	Master	GPA	Work Exp	Letters	Interview
M	Community Counseling	1	14 14							Y
M	Marriage and Family Counseling		14							Y
M	Rehabilitation Counseling		14							Y
M	School Counseling		14							Y

Graduation Requirements

Degree	Program	Academic Hours Sem Qtr	Clock Hours Pract Intern	Thesis	Comp	Examinations CPCE	Oral	Portfolio
M	Community Counseling	72	100 600		Y			Y
M	Marriage and Family Counseling	72	100 600		Y			
M	Rehabilitation Counseling	72	100 600		Y			
M	School Counseling	72	100 600		Y			

OR: Southern Oregon University

1250 Siskiyou Blvd
Ashland, OR 97520
United States of America
http://www.sou.edu/psychology/mhc

Dean   Alyssa Arp
                     College of Arts and Sciences
                     1250 Siskiyou Blvd
                     CS 211
                     Ashland, OR 97520
                     United States of America

Administrator   Josie Wilson, Master in Mental Health Counseling Coordinator
                     1250 Siskiyou Blvd
                     Ed/Psych 222
                     Ashland, OR 97520
                     United States of America
                     (541) 552-6946; fax: (541) 552-6988
                     jwilson@sou.edu

CSI Chapter, Name   N
Regionally Accredited Y
Financial Aid   Y

Satellite Campus: N
International Students: N
Number of International Students: 0

Program Uniqueness

SOU mental health counseling is designated as a Western Regional Graduate Program (WRGP) that allows out-of-state students from the other 14 Western states (Alaska, Arizona, California, Colorado, Hawaii, Idaho, Montana, Nevada, New Mexico, North Dakota, South Dakota, Utah, Washington and Wyoming) to pay in-state tuition. The MHC faculty awards this financial aid to increase diversity and recognize academic excellence. An out-of-state student who would like to be considered for a WRGP award must submit a 300-word essay that addresses how he/she meets one or both of the criteria (diversity and/or academic excellence).

Faculty Research

Counselor education, evidence-based practice, ethical-decision making, school bullying, classroom management, domestic violence in Mexican and Latino families and humanistic psychotherapy.

% faculty in professional counseling practice: NP

Program Accreditation

CACREP: Mental Health Counseling

Degree Programs

Degree	Program	Contact
MS	Mental Health Counseling	Lori Courtney

Distance learning: N; 0% courses on-line

Other Counseling Related Programs
NP

Faculty and Student Ethnicity

Faculty	Master's	Specialist	Doctoral
Asian-American	Asian-American		
Caucasian	Caucasian		
	Latino/Latina		
	Other		

Faculty

Name			Highest Degree	Rank	Time	Credentials State Lic.	NCC	Email
Fujitsubo	Lani	C	PhD	Full Professor	41-60		N	fujitsubo@sou.edu
Kyle	Patricia	B	PhD	Associate Professor	41-60	Y	N	kylep@sou.edu
Murray	Paul	D	PhD	Full Professor	61-80		N	murray@sou.edu
Pierson	J. Fraser		PhD	Full Professor	41-60	N	Y	pierson@sou.edu
Smith	Douglas		PhD	Associate Professor	22-40		N	SmithDou@sou.edu
Wilson	Josie	A	PhD	Full Professor	41-60		N	jwilson@sou.edu

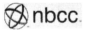   Percent of faculty with NCC certification: 16%

Other Credentials Held By Faculty Members: Certified School Counselor, Certified School Psychologist, Licensed Psychologist

Enrollment and Admission Requirements

Degree	Program	Gender F	M	Yearly Admit	Grad	GRE Total	MAT	Master	GPA	Work Exp	Letters	Interview
MS	Mental Health Counseling	16	6	22	20	1000		Y	3		3	N

Graduation Requirements

Degree	Program	Academic Hours Sem	Qtr	Clock Hours Pract	Intern	Thesis	Examinations Comp	CPCE	Oral	Portfolio
MS	Mental Health Counseling	0	92	100	900	N	N	Y	N	Y

PA: Biblical Seminary

200 N. Main Street
Hatfield, PA 19440
United States of America
www.biblical.edu

Dean

R. Todd Mangum, Dean of Faculty
200 N. Main Street
Hatfield, PA 19440
United States of America

Administrator

Philip G. Monroe
Associate Professor of Counseling & Psychology
Director of MA in Counseling Program
200 N. Main Street
Hatfield, PA 19440
United States of America
(215) 368-5000 x142; fax: NP
pmonroe@biblical.edu

CSI Chapter, Name N
Regionally Accredited Y
Financial Aid Y

Satellite Campus: N
International Students: Y
Number of International Students: 20

Program Uniqueness

Seminary-based professional counseling and Christian psychology program. Delivered in a cohort format with courses offered one night per week and one Saturday per month. Designed for adult learners. Postgraduate advanced counseling certificate. On-site counseling center. Large database of fieldwork placements. Fieldwork director and student liaison on staff give regular student support in program and in placements. All faculty and adjuncts maintain active counseling case loads.

Faculty Research

Forgiveness; history and philosophy of psychology; sexual abuse and addiction; Christian psychology; play therapy.

100% faculty in professional counseling practice.

Degree Programs

Degree	Program	Contact
MA	Counseling	Philip G. Monroe, PsyD

Distance learning: Y; 20% courses on-line

Other Counseling Related Programs

CAPC- Certificate in Advanced Professional Counseling
M.A. in Ministry with Counseling Concentration

Faculty and Student Ethnicity

Faculty	Master's	Specialist	Doctoral
Caucasian	African-American		
	Asian		
	Asian-American		
	Caucasian		
	Latino/Latina		

Faculty

Name			Highest Degree	Rank	Time	Credentials State Lic.	NCC	Email
Altringer	Michelle	L	MA	Adjunct	22-40	N	N	maltringer@biblical.edu
Lowe	Julie	S	MA	Adjunct	<21	Y	N	jlowe@ccef.org
Maier	Bryan	N	PsyD	Associate Professor	>81		N	bmaier@biblical.edu
Monroe	Philip	G	PsyD	Associate Professor and Chair	61-80		N	pmonroe@biblical.edu
Steich	Bonnie	M	MA	Adjunct	<21	N	N	bsteich@biblical.edu
Zuck	Jennifer	A	MA	Adjunct	22-40	N	N	JZuck@biblical.edu

Percent of faculty with NCC certification: 0%

Other Credentials Held By Faculty Members: Licensed Psychologist, LPC

Enrollment and Admission Requirements

Degree	Program	Gender		Yearly		GRE	MAT	Master	GPA	Work	Letters	Interview
		F	M	Admit	Grad	Total				Exp		
MA	Counseling	12	8	25	20			Y			2	Y

Graduation Requirements

Degree	Program	Academic Hours		Clock Hours				Examinations			
		Sem	Qtr	Pract	Intern	Thesis	Comp	CPCE	Oral	Portfolio	
MA	Counseling	52		100	600	N	Y	N	N	Y	

PA: California University of Pennsylvania

250 University Avenue, Box 13
California, PA 15419-1394
United States of America
http://www.calu.edu

Dean

John Cencich, Interim Dean
School of Graduate Studies and Research
250 University Avenue/Box 91
California University of PA
California, PA 15419-4123
United States of America

Administrator

Jacqueline A. Walsh, Ph.D., Chairperson
250 University Avenue, Box 13
California, PA 15419-1394
United States of America
(724) 938-4123; fax: (724) 938-4314
walsh@calu.edu

CSI Chapter, Name Y, Beta Gamma Delta
Regionally Accredited Y
Financial Aid Y

Satellite Campus: N
International Students: NP
Number of International Students: NP

Program Uniqueness

1. Program emphasis on self-awareness. We require students to participate in a personal growth group, for credit, that is facilitated by a faculty member outside of the department. This sets the tone - experiential activities are infused throughout the curriculum. 2. Program provides master's degree as required for Pennsylvania professional counseling license. 3. Graduate certificate in sports counseling (100% online).

Faculty Research

Career counseling, college counseling, sports counseling, student affairs, supervision, mind-body issues in counseling, use of technology in counseling.

50% faculty in professional counseling practice.

Program Accreditation

CACREP: Community Counseling; **CACREP:** School Counseling

Degree Programs

Degree	Program	Contact
MS	Community Counseling	Jacqueline A. Walsh, PhD
MEd	School Counseling	Jacqueline A. Walsh, PhD

Distance learning: N; 1% courses on-line

Other Counseling Related Programs

Communications
Psychology
Social Work

Faculty and Student Ethnicity

Faculty	Master's	Specialist	Doctoral
African-American	African-American		
Caucasian	Asian-American		
Multiracial	Caucasian		
Native American	Latino/Latina		
	Multiracial		
	Native American		

Faculty

Name			Highest Degree	Rank	Time	Credentials State Lic.	NCC	Email
Brusoski	Gloria	C	PhD	Professor		N	N	Brusoski@calu.edu
Eliason	Grafton	T	EdD	Associate Professor		Y	Y	Eliason@calu.edu
Gruber	Elizabeth		PhD	Professor		Y	Y	Gruber@calu.edu
John	Pakako		EdD	Professor		Y	Y	john@calu.edu
Samide	Jeff	L	EdD	Associate Professor		Y	Y	samide@calu.edu
Tinsley	Taunya	M	PhD	Assistant Professor		Y	Y	tinsley@calu.edu
Walsh	Jacqueline	A	PhD	Associate Professor and Chair		Y	Y	walsh@calu.edu

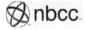 Percent of faculty with NCC certification: 86%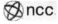

Other Credentials Held By Faculty Members: Approved Clinical Supervisor, CRC, CSC, Licensed Psychologist, LPC

Enrollment and Admission Requirements

Degree	Program	Gender F	M	Yearly Admit	Grad	GRE Total	MAT	Master	GPA	Work Exp	Letters	Interview
MS	Community Counseling	38	9	15	15	0	403	Y	3		3	Y
MEd	School Counseling	31	8	18	13	0	403	Y	3		3	Y

Graduation Requirements

Degree	Program	Academic Hours Sem	Qtr	Clock Hours Pract	Intern	Thesis	Examinations Comp	CPCE	Oral	Portfolio
MS	Community Counseling	48		150	600	N	Y	Y	N	N
MEd	School Counseling	48		150	600		Y	Y		

PA: Gannon University

Community Counseling Program
Department of Psychology and Counseling
109 University Square
Erie, PA 16541-0001
United States of America
www.gannon.edu/communitycounseling

Dean   Tim Downs, Dean of the College of Humanities, Education and Social Sciences
Community Counseling Program
Department of Psychology and Counseling
109 University Square
Erie, PA 16541-0001
United States of America

Administrator   Ken McCurdy, Program Director
Community Counseling Program
Gannon University
109 University Square
Erie, PA 16541-0001
United States of America
(814) 871-7791; fax: (814) 871-5511
mccurdy003@gannon.edu

CSI Chapter, Name   Y, Gamma Upsilon Chi
Regionally Accredited Y
Financial Aid   Y

Satellite Campus: N
International Students: N
Number of International Students: 0

Program Uniqueness

The Master's program in Community Counseling began in 1966. It has a long history of preparing
counseling professionals for practice and advanced training. The program emphasizes a
professional counselor identity, and incorporates ACA, CACREP, PCA, and other counseling
organization standards into the curriculum. Students are prepared to qualify for the National
Certified Counselor (NCC) credential and state licensure as an LPC.

Faculty Research

Cognitive-behavioral therapy; Adlerian counseling; relaxation training; counseling and spirituality;
child, adolescent and family counseling; play therapy; crisis and disaster counseling; legal and
ethical issues in counseling; multicultural issues in counseling; counseling pedagogy;
bereavement issues in counseling; counseling outcome research; hope theory; assessment,
diagnosis and treatment planning; technology in counseling; counselor supervision.

25% faculty in professional counseling practice.

Program Accreditation

CACREP: Community Counseling

Degree Programs

Degree	Program	Contact
M	Community Counseling	Kenneth McCurdy
Advanced Graduate Certificate	Post Graduate Certificate Programs	Kenneth McCurdy

Distance learning: N; 0% courses on-line

Other Counseling Related Programs
NP

Faculty and Student Ethnicity

Faculty	Master's	Specialist	Doctoral
Caucasian	African-American	Caucasian	
	Asian-American		
	Caucasian		
	Latino/Latina		

Faculty

Name			Highest Degree	Rank	Time	Credentials State Lic.	NCC	Email
Coppock	Timothy		PhD	Assistant Professor	61-80	Y	Y	coppock001@gannon.edu
McCurdy	Kenneth	G	PhD	Associate Professor	61-80	Y	Y	mccurdy003@gannon.edu
Tobin	David		PhD	Associate Professor	61-80	N	Y	tobin001@gannon.edu
Willow	Rebecca	A	EdD	Associate Professor	61-80	Y	Y	willow004@gannon.edu

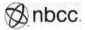   Percent of faculty with NCC certification: 100%

Other Credentials Held By Faculty Members: ACS, Certified Elementary School Counselor, LMHC, LPC, LPC Supervisor, PCC

Enrollment and Admission Requirements

Degree	Program	Gender F	M	Yearly Admit	Grad	GRE Total	MAT	Master	GPA	Work Exp	Letters	Interview
M	Community Counseling	50	10	20	18	0		Y	2.8	1	3	Y
Advanced Graduate Certificate	Post Graduate Certificate Programs	5	2	5	5	0		Y	3			Y

Graduation Requirements

Degree	Program	Academic Hours Sem	Qtr	Clock Hours Pract	Intern	Examinations Thesis	Comp	CPCE	Oral	Portfolio
M	Community Counseling	60		100	600	N	Y	Y		Y
Advanced Graduate Certificate	Post Graduate Certificate Programs	12		100	600	N	N	N	N	N

PA: Messiah College

1 College Avenue
Grantham, PA 17027
United States of America
www.messiah.edu/counseling

Dean

Susan Hasseler, Ph.D.
Dean of the School of Business, Education and Social Sciences
1 College Avenue
Box 3045
Grantham, PA 17027
United States of America

Administrator

John Addleman, Director of the Graduate Program in Counseling
1 College Avenue
Box 3052
Grantham, PA 17027
United States of America
(717) 796-1800, ext. 2980; fax: (717) 691-2386
JAddlemn@messiah.edu

CSI Chapter, Name   N
Regionally Accredited   Y
Financial Aid   Y

Satellite Campus: N
International Students: N
Number of International Students: 0

Program Uniqueness

M.A. in counseling with concentrations in mental health counseling; marriage, couple and family counseling; or school counseling. Courses offered primarily online in 8-week sessions. Two residential one-week intensive courses required. Rolling admissions.

Faculty Research
NP

% faculty in professional counseling practice: NP

Degree Programs

Degree	Program	Contact
MA	Marriage, Couple and Family Counseling	Dr. John Addleman
MA	Mental Health Counseling	Dr. John Addleman
MA	School Counseling	Dr. John Addleman

Distance learning: Y; 98% courses on-line

Other Counseling Related Programs
NP

Faculty and Student Ethnicity
NP

Faculty
NP

Percent of faculty with NCC certification: NP

Other Credentials Held By Faculty Members
NP

Enrollment and Admission Requirements

Degree	Program	Gender		Yearly		GRE	MAT	Master	GPA	Work	Letters	Interview
		F	M	Admit	Grad	Total				Exp		
MA	Marriage, Couple, and Family Counseling					0		Y	3		2	Y
MA	Mental Health Counseling					0		Y	3		2	Y
MA	School Counseling					0		Y	3		2	Y

Graduation Requirements

Degree	Program	Academic Hours		Clock Hours		Examinations				
		Sem	Qtr	Pract	Intern	Thesis	Comp	CPCE	Oral	Portfolio
MA	Marriage, Couple, and Family Counseling	60		100	600	N	Y	Y	N	Y
MA	Mental Health Counseling	60		100	600	N	Y	Y	N	Y
MA	School Counseling	51		100	600	N	N	N	N	Y

PA: Penn State University

307 CEDAR Building
University Park, PA 16802
United States of America
http://www.ed.psu.edu/educ/cecprs/counselor-educatio

Dean
David Monk, Dean
College of Education
274 Chambers Building
University Park, PA 16802

Administrator
Richard Hazler, NCC, PCC, Professor-in-charge
307 CEDAR Building
University Park, PA 16802
United States of America
(814) 865-3428; fax: (814) 863-7750
hazler@psu.edu

CSI Chapter, Name   Y, Rho Alpha Mu
Regionally Accredited Y
Financial Aid   NP

Satellite Campus: N
International Students: Y
Number of International Students: 5

Program Uniqueness

Most students in the program are full time. Faculty members take a mentoring approach to working with students. Students are actively involved in program development and program activities. The program has a rich history of leadership in the profession and the faculty is committed to continual program development. The program is consistently ranked in the top 10 counselor education programs nationwide.

Faculty Research

Several faculty are leading career development researchers. Other faculty interests include school counseling, multicultural topics and rehabilitation topics.

% faculty in professional counseling practice: NP

Program Accreditation

CACREP: Counselor Education and Supervision; **CACREP:** School Counseling; **CORE:** Rehabilitation Counseling

CACREP

Degree Programs

Degree	Program	Contact
M	Rehabilitation Counseling	
M	School Counseling	
PhD	Counselor Education	

Distance learning: NP; % courses on-line: NP

Other Counseling Related Programs
NP

Faculty and Student Ethnicity

Faculty	Master's	Specialist	Doctoral
African-American			
Caucasian			

Faculty

Name			Highest Degree	Rank	Time	Credentials State Lic.	NCC	Email
Bieschke	Kathleen		PhD				N	
Carney	Jolynn		PhD			Y	N	
Conyers	Liza		PhD				N	
Hayes	Jeffrey		PhD				N	
Hazler	Richard		PhD			Y	Y	
Herbert	James		PhD			Y	N	
Herr	Edwin	L	EdD		>81	Y	Y	
Hunt	Brandon		PhD			Y	N	
Mellin	Elizabeth		PhD			Y	N	
Niles	Spencer	G	EdD		>81	Y	Y	
O'Sullivan	Deidre		PhD				N	
Skowran	Elizabeth		PhD				N	
Trusty	Jerry		PhD		>81	Y	Y	
Wilson	Keith		PhD				N	
Woodhouse	Susan		PhD				N	

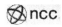

Percent of faculty with NCC certification: 27%

Other Credentials Held By Faculty Members: NP

Enrollment and Admission Requirements

Degree	Program	Gender F	M	Yearly Admit	Grad	GRE Total	MAT	Master	GPA	Work Exp	Letters	Interview
M	Rehabilitation Counseling											
M	School Counseling											
PhD	Counselor Education											

Graduation Requirements

Degree	Program	Academic Hours			Clock Hours			Examinations			
		Sem	Qtr	Pract	Intern	Thesis	Comp	CPCE	Oral	Portfolio	
M	Rehabilitation Counseling										
M	School Counseling										
PhD	Counselor Education										

PA: Shippensburg University of PA

1871 Old Main Drive
Shippensburg, PA 17257-2299
United States of America
www.ship.edu/~counsel

Dean   James Johnson, Ph.D.
1871 Old Main Drive
Shippensburg University, PA 17257
United States of America

Administrator   Jan Arminio, Ph.D., Chairperson
1871 Old Main Drive
Shippensburg, PA 17257-2299
United States of America
(717) 477-1668; fax: (717) 477-4056
jlarmi@ship.edu

CSI Chapter, Name   Y, NP
Regionally Accredited Y
Financial Aid   Y

Satellite Campus: N
International students: Y
Number of International students: 2

Program Uniqueness

All teaching faculty have extensive experience as practitioners. We emphasize authentic relationships with invested faculty who model intentional practice based firmly in theory and cultural advocacy. Students develop knowledge and skills necessary to be purposeful and effective practitioners with a strong sense of personal and professional identity.

Faculty Research

Adolescence, substance abuse and group counseling.

50% faculty in professional counseling practice.

Program Accreditation

CACREP: College Counseling; **CACREP:** Community Counseling; **CACREP:** Mental Health Counseling; **CACREP:** School Counseling; **CACREP:** Student Affairs

Degree Programs

Degree	Program	Contact
M	College Counseling	A. A. Hess
M	Mental Health Counseling	W. W. Brooks
M	School Counseling	Thomas Hozman
M	Student Affairs	Thomas Hozman

Distance learning: N; 10% courses on-line

Other Counseling Related Programs
NP

Faculty and Student Ethnicity

Faculty	**Master's**	**Specialist**	**Doctoral**
African-American	African-American		
Caucasian	Asian-American		
	Caucasian		
	Latino/Latina		
	Multiracial		
	Native American		
	Pacific Islander		

Faculty

Name			Highest Degree	Rank	Time	Credentials State Lic.	NCC	Email
Arminio	Jan	L	PhD	Associate Professor	>81		N	jlarmi@ship.edu
Brooks	Clifford	W	EdD	Associate Professor	>81	Y	Y	cwbroo@ship.edu
Carey	Andrew	L	PhD	Assistant Professor	>81		Y	alcare@ship.edu
Hess	Shirley	A	PhD	Assistant Professor	>81	Y	Y	sahess@ship.edu
Hozman	Thomas	L	PhD	Full Professor	>81		N	tlhozm@ship.edu
Kraus	Kurt	L	EdD	Assistant Professor	>81	Y	Y	klkrau@ship.edu
Kurdt	Kathryn	A	PhD	Assistant Professor	<21	Y	N	kakurd@ship.edu
LaFountain	Rebecca	M	EdD	Full Professor	>81	Y	Y	rmlafo@ship.edu
Mustaine	Beverly	L	EdD	Full Professor	>81	Y	Y	blmust@ship.edu

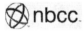   Percent of faculty with NCC certification: 67%

Other Credentials Held By Faculty Members: CAC, CCMHC

Enrollment and Admission Requirements

Degree	Program	Gender F	M	Yearly Admit	Grad	GRE Total	MAT	Master	GPA	Work Exp	Letters	Interview
M	College Counseling	2	2	3	2	800		Y	2.75	1	3	Y
M	Mental Health Counseling	45	5	15	10	800			2.75	1	3	Y
M	School Counseling	83	15	29	20	800			3	1	3	Y
M	Student Affairs	24	9	10	7	800			2.75	1	3	Y

Graduation Requirements

Degree	Program	Academic Hours Sem	Qtr	Clock Hours Pract	Intern	Thesis	Comp	Examinations CPCE	Oral	Portfolio
M	College Counseling	48		150	600	N	N	N	N	Y
M	Mental Health Counseling	60		150	900	N	N	N	N	Y
M	School Counseling	48		150	600					Y
M	Student Affairs	48		150	600					Y

PA: Slippery Rock University

Department of Counseling and Development
006 McKay Education Building
Slippery Rock, PA 16057
United States of America
http://www.sru.edu/pages/4974.asp

Dean NP

Administrator NP

CSI Chapter, Name Y, Alpha Gamma
Regionally Accredited Y
Financial Aid Y

Satellite Campus: N
International students: Y
Number of International students: 1

Program Uniqueness
NP

Faculty Research
NP

% faculty in professional counseling practice: NP

Program Accreditation

CACREP: Community Counseling; **CACREP:** School Counseling; **CACREP:** Student Affairs

Degree Programs

Degree	*Program*	*Contact*
	Community Counseling	Dr. Donald A. Strano

Distance learning: N; 0% courses on-line

Other Counseling Related Programs
NP

Faculty and Student Ethnicity
NP

Faculty
NP

Percent of faculty with NCC certification: NP

Other Credentials Held By Faculty Members: NP

Enrollment and Admission Requirements

Degree	Program	Gender F	M	Yearly Admit	Grad	GRE Total	MAT	Master	GPA	Work Exp	Letters	Interview
	Community Counseling			L1	1							

Graduation Requirements

Degree	Program	Academic Hours Sem	Qtr	Clock Hours Pract	Intern	Thesis	Examinations Comp	CPCE	Oral	Portfolio
	Community Counseling									

SC: Clemson University

313 Tillman Hall, Box 340710
Clemson, SC 29634-0710
United States of America
http://www.clemson.edu/hehd/departments/education/

Dean   Larry Allen
                        College of HEHD

Administrator   Tony W. Cawthon, Professor and Program Chair
                        313 Tillman Hall, Box 340710
                        Clemson, SC 29634-0710
                        United States of America
                        (864) 656-3484; fax: (864) 656-1332
                        cowthot@clemson.edu

CSI Chapter, Name   Y, Chi Upsilon
Regionally Accredited Y
Financial Aid   Y

Satellite Campus: Y
International Students: Y
Number of International Students: 1

Program Uniqueness

Link theory to practice, part-time/full-time students, commitment to multicultural issues and field experience.

Faculty Research

Career development, supervision, multicultural issues, technology, administration, psychopathology, at-risk youth, disabilities, counselor preparation.

% faculty in professional counseling practice: NP

Program Accreditation

CACREP: College Counseling; **CACREP:** Community Counseling; **CACREP:** School Counseling; **CACREP:** Student Affairs

Degree Programs

Degree	Program	Contact
M	College Counseling	Dr. David Scott
M	Community Counseling	Amy Milsom
MEd	School Counseling	
M	Student Affairs	

Distance learning: N; 5% courses on-line

Other Counseling Related Programs

Psychology

Faculty and Student Ethnicity

Faculty	Master's	Specialist	Doctoral
African-American	African-American		
Caucasian	Caucasian		
	Latino/Latina		
	Multiracial		

Faculty

Name		Highest Degree	Rank	Time	Credentials State Lic.	NCC	Email
Abernathy	Larry	M		>81		N	alarry@clemson.edu
Cawthon	Tony	PhD	Professor and Chair			N	cawthot@clemson.edu
Frazier	Kimberly	PhD	Assistant Professor		Y	Y	kfrazie@clemson.edu
Havice	Pamela	PhD	Associate Professor			N	havice@clemson.edu
Hiott	Elaine	M	Clinical Faculty			N	ehiott@clemson.edu
Jerry	Neal	EdD	Instructor		Y	Y	jeromen@clemson.edu
Milsom	Amy	EdD	Associate Professor		Y	Y	amilsom@clemson.edu
Scott	David	PhD	Assistant Professor		Y	N	dscott2@clemson.edu
Warner	Cheryl	PhD	Assistant Professor			N	cforkne@clemson.edu

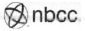 Percent of faculty with NCC certification: 55%

Other Credentials Held By Faculty Members: CDFI, Certified School Counselor, Licensed Psychologist, LMFT, LPC, LPC Supervisor

Enrollment and Admission Requirements

Degree	Program	Gender F	M	Yearly Admit	Grad	GRE Total	MAT	Master	GPA	Work Exp	Letters	Interview
M	College Counseling	4	1	5	2	1250		Y	3		2	Y
M	Community Counseling	20	5	25	25	1000		Y	3		2	
MEd	School Counseling	20	5	25	25	1000			3		2	
M	Student Affairs	20	10	30	20	1250			3		2	

Graduation Requirements

Degree	Program	Academic Hours Sem	Qtr	Clock Hours Pract	Intern	Thesis	Comp	Examinations CPCE	Oral	Portfolio
M	College Counseling	48		100	600		Y	Y		
M	Community Counseling	60		150	600	N	Y	N		
MEd	School Counseling	60		100	600	N	Y	N		
M	Student Affairs	48		100	600		Y			

SC: Webster University

8911 Farrow Road Suite 101
Columbia, SC 29203
United States of America
www.webster.edu/columbia

Dean   Director John Simpson
8911 Farrow Road, Suite 101
Columbia, SC 29203
United States of America

Administrator   NP

CSI Chapter, Name   N
Regionally Accredited Y
Financial Aid   Y

Satellite Campus: N
International Students: Y
Number of International Students: NP

Program Uniqueness

Courses are taught by highly credentialed practitioners, such as LPCs, LPC Supervisors, LMFTs and/or LMFT Supervisors. Students attend classes one time per week for four hours. This typically appeals to the non-traditional working adult student. Each term is nine weeks, and there are five terms in a year.

Faculty Research: NP

% faculty in professional counseling practice: NP

Degree Programs

Degree	*Program*	*Contact*
MA	Master of Arts in Professional Counseling	

Distance learning: N; 0% courses on-line

Other Counseling Related Programs
NP

Faculty and Student Ethnicity
NP

Faculty
NP

Percent of faculty with NCC certification: NP

Other Credentials Held By Faculty Members
NP

Enrollment and Admission Requirements

Degree	Program	Gender F	M	Yearly Admit	Grad	GRE Total	MAT	Master	GPA	Work Exp	Letters	Interview
MA	Master of Arts in Professional Counseling							Y	2.5		3	Y

Graduation Requirements

Degree	Program	Academic Hours Sem	Qtr	Clock Hours Pract	Intern	Thesis	Comp	Examinations CPCE	Oral	Portfolio
MA	Master of Arts in Professional Counseling	60		100	600	N	N	Y	N	N

SD: South Dakota State University

Box 507 Wenona Hall
Brookings, SD 57007-0095
United States of America
www3.sdstate.edu

Dean
Kevin Kephardt
Box 2201 Admin Building
SDSU
Brookings, SD 57007
United States of America

Administrator
Jay Trenhaile, Department Head
Box 507 Wenona Hall
Brookings, SD 57007-0095
United States of America
(605) 688-4190; fax: (605) 688-5929

CSI Chapter, Name   NP
Regionally Accredited   Y
Financial Aid   Y

Satellite Campus: Y
International Students: Y
Number of International Students: 5

Program Uniqueness
NP

Faculty Research

Solution-focused therapy (school and student affairs applications), working with Native American clients and students, and grief counseling.

28% faculty in professional counseling practice.

Program Accreditation

CACREP: College Counseling; **CACREP:** Community Counseling; **CACREP:** School Counseling; **CORE:** Rehabilitation Counseling

Degree Programs

Degree	Program	Contact
M	Community Counseling	Mark Britzman
MS	Rehabilitation Counseling	Alan Davis
M	School Counseling	Hande Briddick
M	Student Affairs	Ruth Harper

Distance learning: Y; 10% courses on-line

Other Counseling Related Programs
NP

Faculty and Student Ethnicity

Faculty	Master's	Specialist	Doctoral
	African-American		
	Caucasian		
	Multiracial		
	Native American		

Faculty

Name		Highest Degree	Rank	Time	Credentials State Lic.	NCC	Email
Briddick	William	PhD	Assistant Professor	>81		Y	William_Briddick@sdstate.edu
Briddick	Hande	PhD	Associate Professor		N	Y	Hande_Briddick@sdstate.edu
Britzman	Mark	EdD	Professor		N	Y	Mark_Britzman@sdstate.edu
Davis	Alan	PhD	Professor	>81	Y	N	Alan.Davis@sdstate.edu
Harper	Ruth	PhD	Professor			Y	Ruth_Harper@sdstate.edu
Muxen	Marla	PhD	Professor		N	N	Marla_Muxen@sdstate.edu
Trenhaile	Jay	EdD	Professor and Chair	<21	N	N	jay.trenhaile@sdstate.edu

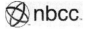 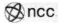

Percent of faculty with NCC certification: 57%

Other Credentials Held By Faculty Members: Approved Clinical Supervisor, Certified School Counselor, Certified School Psychologist, CRC, Licensed Psychologist, Licensed School Counselor

Enrollment and Admission Requirements

Degree	Program	Gender F M	Yearly Admit	Grad	GRE Total	MAT	Master	GPA	Work Exp	Letters	Interview
M	Community Counseling		15	13			Y	3		2	Y
MS	Rehabilitation Counseling		5	4			Y	3		2	Y
M	School Counseling		15	14			Y	3		2	Y
M	Student Affairs		10	9			Y	3		2	Y

Graduation Requirements

Degree	Program	Academic Hours Sem Qtr	Clock Hours Pract	Intern	Examinations Thesis	Comp	CPCE	Oral	Portfolio
M	Community Counseling	48	100	600	N	Y	Y	Y	N
MS	Rehabilitation Counseling	48	100	600	N	Y	Y	Y	N
M	School Counseling	48	100	600	N	Y	Y	Y	N
M	Student Affairs	48	100	600	N	N	Y	Y	N

TN: Argosy University, Nashville

100 Centerview Drive, Suite 225
Nashville, TN 37214
United States of America

Dean NP

Administrator Kittie M. Myatt
Chair, Counselor Education Programs

CSI Chapter, Name NP
Regionally Accredited NP
Financial Aid NP

Satellite Campus: NP
International Students: NP
Number of International Students: NP

Program Uniqueness
NP

Faculty Research
NP

% faculty in professional counseling practice: NP

Degree Programs
NP

Distance learning: NP; % courses on-line: NP

Other Counseling Related Programs
NP

Faculty and Student Ethnicity
NP

Faculty
NP

Percent of faculty with NCC certification: NP

Other Credentials Held By Faculty Members
NP

Enrollment and Admission Requirements
NP

Graduation Requirements
NP

TN: Freed Hardeman University

158 East Main Street
Henderson, TN 38340
United States of America

Dean   Steve Johnson
158 East Main Street
Henderson, TN 38340
United States of America

Administrator   Mike Cravens, Director of M.S. in Counseling
158 East Main Street
Henderson, TN 38340
United States of America
(731) 989-6666; fax: (731) 989-6679
mcravens@fhu.edu

CSI Chapter, Name   N
Regionally Accredited Y
Financial Aid   Y

Satellite Campus: Y
International Students: Y
Number of International Students: 2

Program Uniqueness
NP

Faculty Research
NP

90% faculty in professional counseling practice.

Program Accreditation
NP

Degree Programs
NP

Distance learning: N; 0% courses on-line

Other Counseling Related Programs
NP

Faculty and Student Ethnicity
NP

Faculty
NP

Percent of faculty with NCC certification: NP

Other Credentials Held By Faculty Members
NP

Enrollment and Admission Requirements
NP

Graduation Requirements
NP

TN: Lipscomb University

One University Park Drive
Nashville, TN 37204
United States of America
http://counseling.lipscomb.edu/

Dean   Norma Burgess
Dean of the School of Arts and Sciences
One University Park Drive
Nashville, TN 37204
United States of America

Administrator   Jake Morris
Director of Graduate Programs in Psychology and Counseling
Ward 156
One University Park Drive
Nashville TN, 37204
United States of America
(615) 966-6652; fax: (615) 966-7073
jake.morris@lipscomb.edu

CSI Chapter, Name   N
Regionally Accredited Y
Financial Aid   Y

Satellite Campus: N
International Students: Y
Number of International Students: 4

Program Uniqueness
NP

Faculty Research
NP

% faculty in professional counseling practice: NP

Degree Programs
NP

Distance learning: N; 20% courses on-line

Other Counseling Related Programs
NP

Faculty and Student Ethnicity
NP

Faculty
NP

Percent of faculty with NCC certification: NP

Other Credentials Held By Faculty Members
NP

Enrollment and Admission Requirements
NP

Graduation Requirements
NP

TN: Pentecostal Theological Seminary

900 Walker St.
Cleveland, TN 37311
United States of America
www.ptseminary.edu

Dean   NP
Pentcostal Theological Seminary
900 Walker St.
Cleveland, TN 37311
United States of America

Administrator   Oliver McMahan, Coordinator of the Master of Arts in Counseling
Pentcostal Theological Seminary
900 Walker St.
Cleveland, TN 37311
United States of America
(423) 478-7037; fax: (423) 478-7519
omcmahan@ptseminary.edu

CSI Chapter, Name   N
Regionally Accredited Y
Financial Aid   Y

Satellite Campus: N
International Students: Y
Number of International Students: 2

Program Uniqueness
NP

Faculty Research
NP

% faculty in professional counseling practice: NP

Degree Programs

Degree	*Program*	*Contact*
MA	Mental Health Counseling	

Distance learning: Y; 40% courses on-line

Other Counseling Related Programs
NP

Faculty and Student Ethnicity

Faculty	**Master's**	**Specialist**	**Doctoral**
Pacific Islander	African-American		
	Asian		
	Asian-American		
	Latino/Latina		
	Multiracial		

Faculty

Name			Highest Degree	Rank	Time	Credentials State Lic.	NCC	Email
Biller	Tom		EdD	Assistant Professor	22-40	Y	N	
McMahan	Oliver	L		Full Professor	22-40	N	N	omcmahan@ptseminary.edu
Queen	Luke		DSc	Adjunct	22-40	Y	Y	lukequeen@gmail.com
Slocumb	Douglas	W	DMin	Associate Professor	22-40		N	dslocumb@ptseminary.edu
Vining	John	K	DMin	Adjunct	22-40	Y	N	

 Percent of faculty with NCC certification: 20%

Other Credentials Held By Faculty Members: Licensed Psychologist, LMFT, LMHC

Enrollment and Admission Requirements

Degree	Program	Gender F	M	Yearly Admit	Grad	GRE Total	MAT	Master	GPA	Work Exp	Letters	Interview
MA	Mental Health Counseling	20	20	10	6							

Graduation Requirements

Degree	Program	Academic Hours Sem	Qtr	Clock Hours Pract	Intern	Thesis	Comp	Examinations CPCE	Oral	Portfolio
MA	Mental Health Counseling									

TN: Psychological Studies Institute

1815 McCallie Avenue
Chattanooga, TN 37404
United States of America
www.psy.edu

Dean   Philip A. Coyle, Academic Dean
1815 McCallie Avenue
Chattanooga, TN 37404
United States of America

Administrator   Cara Cochran, Assistant Academic Dean
1815 McCallie Avenue
Chattanooga, TN 37404
United States of America

CSI Chapter, Name   N
Regionally Accredited Y
Financial Aid   Y

Satellite Campus: NP
International Students: NP
Number of International Students: NP

Program Uniqueness

The Psychological Studies Institute (PSI) provides graduate counselor education, integrating applied psychology and practical theology to make Christian counseling a servant of the church for Christ-centered transformation. Students may obtain an M.A. in Professional Counseling, an M.A. in Marriage and Family Therapy (meets AAMFT standards), or an M.S. in Christian Psychological Studies (not a licensure track degree). PSI offers all of its degree programs in Atlanta and Chattanooga. Students may choose from one of five specializations: addictions counseling, child and adolescent counseling, Christian sex therapy, leadership and coaching, or spirituality and counseling. Our school has fully staffed campuses in Chattanooga and Atlanta. Our students obtain sound clinical skills while learning how to allow their faith to inform their practice. Some of the best known clinicians in the world served as our faculty members, including Gary Collins, David Benner, Gary Moon, Siang-Yang Tan and Doug Rosenau.

Faculty Research

Dr. Jeff Terrell, PSI president: the relationship between mental disorders and religious commitments. Dr. Gary Moon, vice president: spiritual formation and mental health. Dr. Phil Coyle, academic dean: family health and development of family health inventory. Dr. Cara Cochran: theology in counselor education, and reconciliation and implications for counseling. Dr. Tim Sisemore: childhood anxiety, children's spirituality and coping. Dr. Lynne Harris: clergy families and mental health, attachment in supervision. Dr. Jana Pressley: attachment theory and personality development. Dr. Jama White: attachment theory. Dr. Steve Bradshaw: family mantras and forgiveness, and interpersonal healing.

95% faculty in professional counseling practice.

Degree Programs

Degree	Program	Contact
MA	Master of Arts in Marriage and Family Therapy	Jessica Jennings, M.A.
MA	Master of Arts in Professional Counseling	Jessica Jennings, M.A.
MS	Master of Science in Christian Psychological Studies	Jessica Jennings, M.A.

Distance learning: N; % courses on-line: NP

Other Counseling Related Programs
NP

Faculty and Student Ethnicity
NP

Faculty

Name			Highest Degree	Rank	Time	Credentials State Lic.	NCC	Email
Benner	David	G	PhD	Distinguished Professor	<21	N	N	
Bradshaw	Stephen	P	PhD	Adjunct	<21	N	N	
Bunger	Ron		MDiv	Other	<21	N	N	
Cappecchi	Elizabeth		PhD	Adjunct	<21	N	N	
Cochran	Cara		PhD	Assistant Academic Dean & Assistant Professor	<21	Y	N	
Collins	Gary	R	PhD	Other	<21	N	N	
Cooper	David	C	DMin	Adjunct	<21	N	N	
Coyle	Philip	A	PhD	Academic Dean & Professor	22-40	Y	Y	
Deardorff	David	E	EdD	Assistant Professor	<21	Y	N	
Doverspike	William		PhD	Adjunct	<21	N	N	
Eckert	Jeffery	S	PsyD	Assistant Professor	<21	N	N	
Gladson	Jerry	A	PhD	Adjunct	<21		N	
Goehring	Marty		PhD	Adjunct	<21		N	
Hanshew	Evalin	R	PhD	Dean of Clinical Activities & Associate Professor	<21	Y	Y	
Harris	Lynne		PhD	Assistant Dean of Students & Assistant Professor	22-40	N	N	
Hermecz	David	L	PhD	Adjunct	<21		N	
Hughes	John	E	MS	Other	<21		N	
James	J.	W	PsyD	Adjunct	<21		N	
McGee	William	D	EdD	Assistant Professor	<21		N	
Moon	Gary	J	PhD	Other	<21	N	N	
Pressley	Jana		PsyD	Assistant Dean of Students & Assistant Professor	22-40	Y	N	
Reid	Michael	A	PhD	Assistant Professor	22-40		N	
Rosenau	Douglas	M	EdD	Adjunct	<21		N	
Sisemore	Timothy		PhD	Other	<21		N	
Siwy	James	C	PhD	Adjunct	<21		N	
Slocumb	Douglas		DMin	Associate Professor and Chair		Y	N	dslocumb@ptseminary.edu
Snook	Stephen		PhD	Adjunct	<21		N	
Sytsma	Michael	J	PhD	Adjunct	<21		N	
Tan	Siang-	C	PhD	Adjunct	<21		N	
Terrell	YaNg		PhD	Other	<21		N	
Terrell	Deanne		PhD	Other	<21		N	
Tiggleman	Jeffrey		PhD	Assistant Professor	<21		N	
Uomoto	Casey	L	PhD	Adjunct	<21	Y	N	
Walker	Jay Donald		PhD	Director of Institutional Effectiveness & Assistant Professor	22-40		N	
White	Jama		PsyD	Other	<21		Y	

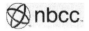   Percent of faculty with NCC certification: 8%

Other Credentials Held By Faculty Members: AAMFT Approved Supervisor, AAMFT Clinical Member, Licensed Psychologist, LMFT, LMFT Supervisor, LPC Supervisor

Enrollment and Admission Requirements

Degree	Program	Gender		Yearly		GRE Total	MAT	Master	GPA	Work Exp	Letters	Interview
		F	M	Admit	Grad							
MA	Master of Arts in Marriage and Family Therapy			45	30	1000		Y	3		5	N
MA	Master of Arts in Professional Counseling			45	30	1000		Y	3		5	
MS	Master of Science in Christian Psychological Studies			10	8	1000		Y	3			

Graduation Requirements

Degree	Program	Academic Hours		Clock Hours			Examinations				
		Sem	Qtr	Pract	Intern	Thesis	Comp	CPCE	Oral	Portfolio	
MA	Master of Arts in Marriage and Family Therapy	77		100	600	N	N	Y	N	N	
MA	Master of Arts in Professional Counseling	66		100	700	N	N	Y	N	N	
MS	Master of Science in Christian Psychological Studies	32				N	N	N	N	N	

TN: University of Tennessee at Chattanooga

615 McCallie Avenue, Dept. 2242
Chattanooga, TN 37403
United States of America
http://www.utc.edu/Academic/CounselingProgram/

Dean

Mary Tanner
615 McCallie Avenue
Dept. 4154, Hunter Hall
Chattanooga, TN 37403
United States of America

Administrator

Valerie Rutledge, Head
615 McCallie Avenue
Department 4154, Hunter Hall
Chattanooga, TN 37403
United States of America

CSI Chapter, Name   Y, Upsilon Theta Chi
Regionally Accredited Y
Financial Aid   Y

Satellite Campus: N
International Students: N
Number of International Students: 0

Program Uniqueness
NP

Faculty Research
NP

0% faculty in professional counseling practice.

Program Accreditation

CACREP

CACREP: Community Counseling; **CACREP:** School Counseling

Degree Programs

Degree	Program	Contact
MEd	Community Counseling	
MEd	School Counseling	

Distance learning: N; 10% courses on-line

Other Counseling Related Programs
NP

Faculty and Student Ethnicity
NP

Faculty

Name		Highest Degree	Rank	Time	Credentials State Lic.	NCC	Email
Gibbs	Kristi	PhD	Assistant Professor		Y	N	
Magnus	Virginia	PhD	Assistant Professor			N	
O'Brien	Elizabeth	PhD	Assistant Professor		N	N	

Percent of faculty with NCC certification: 0%

Other Credentials Held By Faculty Members: Licensed School Counselor, LPC, LPC Supervisor, RPTS

Enrollment and Admission Requirements

Degree	Program	Gender F	M	Yearly Admit	Grad	GRE Total	MAT	Master	GPA	Work Exp	Letters	Interview
MEd	Community Counseling	13	2	15	15							
MEd	School Counseling	13	2	15	15							

Graduation Requirements

Degree	Program	Academic Hours Sem	Qtr	Clock Hours Pract	Intern	Thesis	Comp	Examinations CPCE	Oral	Portfolio
MEd	Community Counseling									
MEd	School Counseling									

TX: Angelo State University

Box 10893, ASU Station
San Angelo, TX 76909
United States of America
www.angelo.edu

Dean   John Miazga

Administrator   David J. Tarver, Assistant Professor
Box 10893, ASU Station
San Angelo, TX 76909
United States of America
(325) 942-2052; fax: (325) 942-2039
david.tarver@angelo.edu

CSI Chapter, Name   NP
Regionally Accredited   Y
Financial Aid   NP

Satellite Campus: NP
International Students: NP
Number of International Students: NP

Program Uniqueness

Public school (K-12) guidance and counseling master's program.

Faculty Research

Learned optimism, self-efficacy and locus of control.

% faculty in professional counseling practice: NP

Degree Programs
NP

Distance learning: NP; % courses on-line: NP

Other Counseling Related Programs
NP

Faculty and Student Ethnicity

Faculty	Master's	Specialist	Doctoral
Caucasian			

Faculty
NP

Percent of faculty with NCC certification: NP

Other Credentials Held By Faculty Members: NP

Enrollment and Admission Requirements
NP

Graduation Requirements
NP

TX: Dallas Baptist University

3000 Mountain Creek Pkwy
Dallas, TX 75211-9299
United States of America
www.dbu.edu/graduate/mac.html

Dean   Mike Williams, Dean, College of Humanities
3000 Mountain Creek Pkwy
Dallas, TX 75211-9299
United States of America

Administrator   Mary Becerril, Ph.D.
Director, M.A. in Counseling Program
3000 Mountain Creek Pkwy
Dallas, TX 75211-9299
United States of America
(214) 333-5265; fax: (214) 333-6819
maryb@dbu.edu

CSI Chapter, Name   NP
Regionally Accredited Y
Financial Aid   Y

Satellite Campus: Y
International Students: Y
Number of International Students: 5

Program Uniqueness

Program offers Christian counseling.

Faculty Research

Play therapy certification.

100% faculty in professional counseling practice.

Degree Programs

Degree	*Program*	*Contact*
MA	Mental Health Counseling	Mary Becerril

Distance learning: N; 2% courses on-line

Other Counseling Related Programs: NP

Faculty and Student Ethnicity

Faculty	Master's	Specialist	Doctoral
African-American	African-American		
Caucasian	Asian-American		
	Caucasian		
	Latino/Latina		

Faculty

Name			Highest Degree	Rank	Time	State Lic.	NCC	Email
						Credentials		
Becerril	Mary		PhD	Full Professor		Y	N	maryb@dbu.edu
Cobern	Keith		PhD	Instructor		Y	N	ktcobern@hotmail.com
Colton	Robert		PhD	Full Professor	22-40		N	bob@dbu.edu
Good	Sharon		MA	Adjunct		Y	N	slgood@wans.net
Hemminger	Wade		EdD	Assistant Professor		Y	N	wade@dbu.edu
Houston	Nancy		MA	Adjunct	<21	Y	N	rhouston@@hotmail.com
Linder	Todd		MA	Instructor	<21	Y	N	tlinder@rapha.info
Mungadze	Jerry		PhD	Instructor			N	mungadzw@msn.com
Shaw	Wynn		MEd	Adjunct		Y	N	wmittledorf@dcac.org
Walker	J	D	MA	Adjunct		N	N	jdonwalker@yahoo.com
Wolf	Shannon	M	PhD	Associate Professor		Y	N	shannonw@dbu.edu

Percent of faculty with NCC certification: 0%

Other Credentials Held By Faculty Members: Licensed Psychologist, LMFT, LPC Supervisor

Enrollment and Admission Requirements

Degree	Program	Gender		Yearly		GRE Total	MAT	Master	GPA	Work Exp	Letters	Interview
		F	M	Admit	Grad							
MA	Mental Health Counseling	75	22	95	50	850			3	0	2	N

Graduation Requirements

Degree	Program	Academic Hours		Clock Hours				Examinations			
		Sem	Qtr	Pract	Intern	Thesis	Comp	CPCE	Oral	Portfolio	
MA	Mental Health Counseling	49		300		N	N	N	N	N	

TX: Our Lady of the Lake University

411 S.W. 24th
San Antonio, TX 78207
United States of America
www.ollusa.edu

Dean
Teresita Aguilar
School of Professional Studies

Administrator
Cullen Grinnan, Chairperson
411 S.W. 24th
San Antonio, TX 78207
United States of America
(210) 434-6711; fax: (210) 431-3927
ctgrinnan@ollusa.edu

CSI Chapter, Name Y, Omega Lambda Lambda
Regionally Accredited Y
Financial Aid Y

Satellite Campus: N
International Students: Y
Number of International Students: 2

Program Uniqueness

Focus on brief, systemic approaches and multiculturalism. Offer specialization in providing services to Spanish-speaking clients.

Faculty Research

Multiculturalism, process and effectiveness of brief therapies.

75% faculty in professional counseling practice.

Degree Programs

Degree	Program	Contact
M	Counseling Psychology	Joan Biever
M	Marriage and Family Counseling	Joan Biever
MEd	School Counseling	Cullen Grinnan

Distance learning: Y; % courses on-line: NP

Other Counseling Related Programs

Clinical Social Workers
Psychology

Faculty and Student Ethnicity

Faculty	Master's	Specialist	Doctoral
Caucasian	African-American		
Latino/Latina	Asian-American		
	Caucasian		
	Latino/Latina		
	Multiracial		
	Native American		

Faculty

Name			Highest Degree	Rank	Time	Credentials State Lic.	NCC	Email
Biever	Joan	L	PhD	Full Professor and Director of Graduate Program	22-40	Y	N	jbiever@ollusa.edu
Bobele	Monte		PhD	Full Professor	41-60		N	bobem@lake.olllusa.edu
González	Cynthia		PhD	Associate Professor	>81		N	gonzcy@lake.ollusa.edu
Grinnan	Cullen	H	PhD	Assistant Professor			N	
O`Donnell	Kristin		MS	Instructor	>81	N	N	klodonnell@ollusa.edu
Pena	Ezequiel		PhD	Assistant Professor	>81	N	N	epena@ollusa.edu
Solorzano	Bernadette		PsyD	Associate Professor	61-80	Y	N	bsolorzano@ollusa.edu

Percent of faculty with NCC certification: 0%

Other Credentials Held By Faculty Members: Licensed Psychologist, LPC, LPC Supervisor, LSSP

Enrollment and Admission Requirements

Degree	Program	Gender F	M	Yearly Admit	Grad	GRE Total	MAT	Master	GPA	Work Exp	Letters	Interview
M	Counseling Psychology	7	3	10	10				2.5		2	Y
M	Marriage and Family Counseling	7	3	10	10			N	2.5		2	Y
MEd	School Counseling			7	7			Y	2.75		2	Y

Graduation Requirements

Degree	Program	Academic Hours Sem	Qtr	Clock Hours Pract	Intern	Thesis	Comp	Examinations CPCE	Oral	Portfolio
M	Counseling Psychology	61		500		N	Y	N	N	N
M	Marriage and Family Counseling	60		500		N	Y	N	N	N
MEd	School Counseling	48		300			Y			

TX: Tarleton State University

TO8020
Stephenville, TX 76402
United States of America
www.tarleton.edu

Dean   Jill Burk, Ph.D.

Administrator   David Weissenburger, Head of Department
T-820
Stephenville, TX 76402
United States of America
(254) 968-9090; fax: (254) 968-1995
weissenburge@tarleton.edu

CSI Chapter, Name N
Regionally Accredited Y
Financial Aid Y

Satellite Campus: Y
International Students: N
Number of International Students: 0

Program Uniqueness

The counseling program at Tarleton began with the purpose of preparing school counselors. The program now offers both M.Ed. and M.S. degrees in counseling psychology, marriage and family counseling and educational psychology.

Faculty Research

Research includes school counseling and guidance, stress management, biofeedback, reality therapy, emotion-based counseling theory, spirituality and counseling, assessment of workplace environment, and disorders of childhood.

50% faculty in professional counseling practice.

Degree Programs

Degree	*Program*	*Contact*
MS	Marriage and Family Counseling	Tom Burdenski
MS	Mental Health Counseling	All faculty
MEd	School Counseling	Albrecht, Duncan, Weissenberger

Distance learning: Y; 25% courses on-line

Other Counseling Related Programs
Counseling Psychology
Experimental Psychology
Educational Psychology

Faculty and Student Ethnicity

Faculty	Master's	Specialist	Doctoral
Caucasian	African-American		
Latino/Latina	Asian-American		
	Caucasian		
	Latino/Latina		
	Multiracial		
	Native American		

Faculty

Name		Highest Degree	Rank	Time	Credentials State Lic.	NCC	Email
Albrecht	Annette	PhD	Full Professor		Y	Y	albrech@tarleton.edu
Burdenski	Tom	PhD	Assistant Professor		Y	N	burdenski@tarleton.edu
Duncan	Linda	EdD	Full Professor	>81	Y	N	duncan@tarleton.edu
Valdez	Diana	PhD	Assistant Professor		Y	N	valdez@tarleton.edu
Weissenburger	David	PhD	Full Professor		N	N	weissenburge@tarleton.edu

nbcc.   Percent of faculty with NCC certification: 20%   ncc.

Other Credentials Held By Faculty Members: Licensed Psychologist, LMFT, LPC, LPC Supervisor, MFT

Enrollment and Admission Requirements

Degree	Program	Gender F	M	Yearly Admit	Grad	GRE Total	MAT	Master	GPA	Work Exp	Letters	Interview
MS	Marriage and Family Counseling	5	5	10	5	850		Y	3			N
MS	Mental Health Counseling	32	18	40	25	850		Y	3			N
MEd	School Counseling	60	15	75	40	850		Y	3			N

Graduation Requirements

Degree	Program	Academic Hours Sem	Qtr	Clock Hours Pract	Intern	Thesis	Comp	Examinations CPCE	Oral	Portfolio
MS	Marriage and Family Counseling	48		90	500	N	Y			
MS	Mental Health Counseling	48		60	300	N	Y	N	N	N
MEd	School Counseling	48		60	300	N	Y	N	N	N

TX: Texas State University-San Marcos

601 S. University Drive
San Marcos, TX 78666
United States of America
www.txstate.edu/clas

Dean   Rosalinda Barrera, Dean of Education

Administrator   Linda E. Homeyer, Program Coordinator
601 S. University Drive
San Marcos, TX 78666
United States of America
(512) 245-2575; fax: (512) 245-8872
LHomeyer@txstate.edu

CSI Chapter, Name   Y, Sigma Tau Sigma
Regionally Accredited   Y
Financial Aid   Y

Satellite Campus: Y
International Students: NP
Number of International Students: NP

Program Uniqueness

Our program has a strong clinical skill component. We also believe in the importance of mentoring students. We have a strong expressive arts offering (play therapy, sandtray therapy and psychodrama methods).

Faculty Research: NP

25% faculty in professional counseling practice.

Program Accreditation

CACREP: Community Counseling; **CACREP:** Marital, Couple and Family Counseling/Therapy; **CACREP:** School Counseling

Degree Programs

Degree	*Program*	*Contact*
M	Community Counseling	John Garcia
M	Marriage and Family Counseling	Colleen Connolly
M	School Counseling	Gail Roaten
M	Student Affairs	Stan Carpenter

Distance learning: N; 0% courses on-line

Other Counseling Related Programs

Health Psychology
Social Work

Faculty and Student Ethnicity

Faculty	Master's	Specialist	Doctoral
Caucasian	African-American		
Latino/Latina	Asian-American		
Multiracial	Caucasian		
	Latino/Latina		
	Multiracial		
	Native American		

Faculty

Name			Highest Degree	Rank	Time	Credentials State Lic.	NCC	Email
Beckenbach	John		PhD	Assistant Professor	>81	Y	Y	JBeckenbach@txstate.edu
Carpenter	Stan		PhD	Chair	22-40		N	Stan@txstate.edu
Connolly	Colleen		PhD	Associate Professor	>81	Y	N	cconnolly@txstate.edu
Fall	Kevin		PhD	Associate Professor	>81	Y	Y	KF22@txstate.edu
Garcia	John	L	PhD	Associate Professor	>81	Y	N	jg12@txstate.edu
Garrison	John		PhD	Assistant Professor	<21	N	N	
Homeyer	Linda	E	PhD	Full Professor and Director of Graduate Program	>81	Y	N	LHomeyer@txstate.edu
Morrison	Mary		PhD	Assistant Professor	>81	Y	N	MMorrison@txstate.edu
Patrick	Shawn		PhD	Assistant Professor	>81	Y	Y	sp27@txstate.edu
Roaten	Gail	V	PhD	Assistant Professor	>81	Y	N	GRoaten@txstate.edu
Schmidt	Eric		PhD	Associate Professor	>81	Y	N	es17@txstate.edu
Wyatt	Carl		PhD	Assistant Professor	<21	Y	N	cw23@swt.edu
Ybanez	Kathy		PhD	Assistant Professor	>81	Y	N	KYbanez@txstate.edu

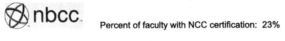

Percent of faculty with NCC certification: 23%

Other Credentials Held By Faculty Members: Certified School Counselor, CSC, LMFT, LMFT Supervisor, LPC, LPC Supervisor, RPTS

Enrollment and Admission Requirements

Degree	Program	Gender F	Gender M	Yearly Admit	Yearly Grad	GRE Total	MAT	Master	GPA	Work Exp	Letters	Interview
M	Community Counseling			20	15	900		Y			3	N
M	Marriage and Family Counseling			30	15	900		Y			3	N
M	School Counseling			15	14	900		Y			3	N
M	Student Affairs	25	5	30	30	900		Y			3	Y

Graduation Requirements

Degree	Program	Academic Hours Sem	Qtr	Clock Hours Pract	Intern	Thesis	Comp	Examinations CPCE	Oral	Portfolio
M	Community Counseling	61		140	600	N	Y	Y	N	N
M	Marriage and Family Counseling	61		140	600	N	Y	Y	N	N
M	School Counseling	55		140	600	N	Y	Y	N	N
M	Student Affairs	48				N	Y	N	Y	N

TX: University of Texas at El Paso

500 W. University Ave.
El Paso, TX 79968
United States of America
www.academics.utep.edu/edpsychology

Dean   Josie Tinajero, Dean, College of Education
University of Texas at El Paso
500 W. University Ave.
El Paso, TX 79968
United States of America

Administrator   Don C. Combs, Ed.D., Department Chair
College of Education
University of Texas at El Paso
500 W. University Ave.
El Paso, TX 79968
United States of America
(915) 747-7585; fax: (915) 747-8410
dcombs@utep.edu

CSI Chapter, Name   Y, Upsilon Tau Epsilon
Regionally Accredited   Y
Financial Aid   Y

Satellite Campus: N
International Students: Y
Number of International Students: 5

Program Uniqueness

We serve a border area multicultural region (Hispanic/Anglo).

Faculty Research

Grief and bereavement counseling, marriage and family counseling, child/adolescent counseling, career counseling, multicultural counseling, crisis counseling, social justice, second language learners, human advocacy, post-traumatic stress and school violence/trauma.

33% faculty in professional counseling practice.

Degree Programs

Degree	*Program*	*Contact*
MEd	Community Counseling	Steve W. Johnson
MEd	School Counseling	Merranda Marin

Distance learning: N; 0% courses on-line

Other Counseling Related Programs

Clinical Psychology
Rehabilitation Counseling
Social Work

Faculty and Student Ethnicity

Faculty	**Master's**	**Specialist**	**Doctoral**
Asian-American	African-American		
Caucasian	Caucasian		
Latino/Latina	Latino/Latina		

Faculty

Name			Highest Degree	Rank	Time	State Lic.	NCC	Email
						Credentials		
Combs	Don	C	EdD	Associate Professor	>81	Y	Y	dcombs@utep.edu
Cortez-Gonzalez	Roberto		PhD	Associate Professor	>81	N	N	rgonzale@utep.edu
Guo	Yuh-Jen		PhD	Assistant Professor	>81	Y	Y	ymguo@utep.edu
Haley	Melinda		PhD	Assistant Professor		N	Y	mahaleybailey2@utep.edu
Johnson	Steve	W	PhD	Associate Professor	>81	Y	N	stevej@utep.edu
Marin	Merranda		PhD	Assistant Professor	>81	N	N	mmarin7@utep.edu

 Percent of faculty with NCC certification: 50%

Other Credentials Held By Faculty Members: CCMHC, Licensed Psychologist, LMFT, LPC, LPC Supervisor

Enrollment and Admission Requirements

Degree	Program	Gender F	Gender M	Yearly Admit	Yearly Grad	GRE Total	MAT	Master	GPA	Work Exp	Letters	Interview
MEd	Community Counseling	10	5	15	15			Y	3.25		3	Y
MEd	School Counseling	12	15	50	50			Y	3.25		3	Y

Graduation Requirements

Degree	Program	Academic Hours Sem	Qtr	Clock Hours Pract	Clock Hours Intern	Thesis	Comp	CPCE	Oral	Portfolio
								Examinations		
MEd	Community Counseling	48		100	600	N	Y	N	N	N
MEd	School Counseling	48		100	600	N	Y	N	N	N

VA: Eastern Mennonite University

Master of Arts in Counseling
1200 Park Road
Harrisonburg, VA 22802
United States of America
www.emu.edu

Dean   P. David Glanzer
Master of Arts in Counseling
1200 Park Road
Harrisonburg, VA 22802
United States of America

Administrator   Annmarie Early
Master of Arts in Counseling
1200 Park Road
Harrisonburg, VA 22802
United States of America
(540) 432-4243; fax: (540) 432-4598
annmarie.early@emu.edu

CSI Chapter, Name   N
Regionally Accredited   Y
Financial Aid   Y

Satellite Campus: N
International Students: N
Number of International Students: 0

Program Uniqueness

Faith-based, experiential training program that trains how to work with intrapersonal and interpersonal dynamics, applying current research on neuroscience and effective processes in creating change, valuing both implicit and explicit modalities.

Faculty Research

Experiential treatment modalities, working experientially in therapy, creativity in counseling, implicit and explicit processes in change, skills acquisition, counselor supervision, marriage and family, grief and widowhood, and ethics.

80% faculty in professional counseling practice

Program Accreditation

CACREP: Community Counseling

Degree Programs

Distance learning: N; % courses on-line: NP

Other Counseling Related Programs

> Center for Justice and Peacebuilding
> Social Work
> Psychology

Faculty and Student Ethnicity

Faculty	**Master's**	**Specialist**	**Doctoral**
	African-American		
	Asian		
	Biracial		
	Latino/Latina		
	Pacific Islander		

Faculty
NP

Percent of faculty with NCC certification: NP

Other Credentials Held By Faculty Members
NP

Enrollment and Admission Requirements
NP

Graduation Requirements
NP

VA: Hampton University

Phenix Hall
Hampton University
Hampton, VA 23668
United States of America
www.hamptonu.edu

Dean
Dean Herring
Phenix Hall
Hampton University
Hampton, VA 23668
United States of America

Administrator
Baker, Coordinator
Phenix Hall
Hampton University
Hampton, VA 23668
United States of America
(757) 727-5128; fax: NP
spencer.baker@hamptonu.edu

CSI Chapter, Name Y, Omega Chi Nu
Regionally Accredited Y
Financial Aid Y

Satellite Campus: N
International Students: N
Number of International Students: 0

Program Uniqueness

The program embraces the holistic person spiritually, mentally, physically and emotionally.

Faculty Research
NP

% faculty in professional counseling practice: NP

Degree Programs
NP

Distance learning: N; 0% courses on-line

Other Counseling Related Programs
NP

Faculty and Student Ethnicity
NP

Faculty
NP

Percent of faculty with NCC certification: NP

Other Credentials Held By Faculty Members
NP

Enrollment and Admission Requirements
NP

Graduation Requirements
NP

VA: James Madison University

MSC 7401
James Madison University
Harrisonburg, VA 22807
United States of America
http://cep.jmu.edu/counselpsyc/

Dean

Sharon Lovell
College of Integrated Science and Technology
James Madison University
Harrisonburg, VA 22807

Administrator

A. Renee Staton, Director
MSC 7401
James Madison University
Harrisonburg, VA 22807
United States of America
(540) 568-7867; fax: (540) 568-4747
statonar@jmu.edu

CSI Chapter, Name   Y, Alpha Sigma
Regionally Accredited   Y
Financial Aid   Y

Satellite Campus: N
International Students: N
Number of International Students: 0

Program Uniqueness

Our philosophy of training is based on five principles: 1) We learn by working together. Our program is a community of learners committed to support one another in the formidable enterprise of becoming a successful counselor. 2) We learn by doing. In virtually every class period, faculty members involve students in some activity that requires them to practice the craft of counseling – the process of observing, gathering information, conceptualizing and taking action. 3) We learn throughout our lives. Counseling professionals have two simple options – to grow as persons and professionals by challenging ourselves or to stagnate. 4) We learn by example. The heart of a counselor education program is not the curriculum, but its people. Actions do speak louder than words, so it is vital that both faculty and students exemplify the values of the counseling profession. 5) When we learn, we change. As students progress through this program, they do more than acquire knowledge and develop skills – they transform themselves professionally and personally.

Faculty Research

Michele Kielty Briggs – school counseling, spirituality, gender, self concept. Eric W. Cowan – self psychology, eating disorders, counseling process; recognized by the JMU Mortarboard for Outstanding Teaching. Lennis G. Echterling – disasters and trauma, brief counseling, crisis intervention; recipient of the national ACES Counseling Vision and Innovation Award, Virginia Outstanding Faculty Award, and the Madison Distinguished Teacher Award. J. Edson McKee – counseling techniques, group dynamics, creativity and learning styles; recipient of the national ACES Professional Service Award, Virginia School Counselor Association Outstanding Counselor Educator Award, and the CISAT Distinguished Teaching Award. Jack H. Presbury – creativity, artificial intelligence, brief therapy, cognitive psychology, history and systems; recipient of the Madison Scholar Award. A. Renee Staton – multicultural issues, community counseling, counselor supervision; past president of the Virginia Counselors Association and the Virginia Association for Counselor Education and Supervision.

88% faculty in professional counseling practice

Program Accreditation

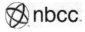

CACREP: Community Counseling; **CACREP**: School Counseling

Degree Programs

Degree	Program	Contact
M	Community Counseling	Sue Rippy
M	School Counseling	Sue Rippy

Distance learning: N; 5% courses on-line

Other Counseling Related Programs
NP

Faculty and Student Ethnicity

Faculty	Master's	Specialist	Doctoral
Caucasian			
Multiracial			

Faculty

Name			Highest Degree	Rank	Time	Credentials State Lic.	NCC	Email
Briggs	Michele	K	PhD	Associate Professor	>81	Y	N	briggsmk@jmu.edu
Cowan	Eric		PsyD	Full Professor	>81		N	cownawe@jmu.edu
Echterling	Lennis	G	PhD	Full Professor	>81		N	echterlg@jmu.edu
McKee	J.E.		EdD	Full Professor		Y	N	mckeeje@jmu.edu
Presbury	Jack	H	EdD	Full Professor	>81	Y	N	presubjh@jmu.edu
Staton	Renee	A	PhD	Associate Professor		Y	Y	statonar@jmu.edu
Stewart	Anne	L	PhD	Full Professor	22-40		N	stewaral@jmu.edu

Percent of faculty with NCC certification: 14%

Other Credentials Held By Faculty Members: Licensed Psychologist

Enrollment and Admission Requirements

Degree	Program	Gender F	M	Yearly Admit	Grad	GRE Total	MAT	Master	GPA	Work Exp	Letters	Interview
M	Community Counseling			10	10							
M	School Counseling			10	10							

Graduation Requirements

Degree	Program	Academic Hours Sem	Qtr	Clock Hours Pract	Intern	Thesis	Comp	Examinations CPCE	Oral	Portfolio
M	Community Counseling	60		100	900					
M	School Counseling	60		100	600					

VA: Marymount University

Department of Counseling
School of Education and Human Services
2807 N. Glebe Road
Arlington, VA 22207
United States of America

Dean   Wayne Lesko
School of Education and Human Services
2807 North Glebe Road
Arlington, VA 22207
United States of America

Administrator   Lisa Jackson-Cherry, Department Chair
Department of Counseling
School of Education and Human Services
2807 North Glebe Road
Arlington, VA 22207
United States of America
(703) 284-5705; fax: (703) 284-1631
www.marymount.edu

CSI Chapter, Name   Y, Mu Upsilon Gamma
Regionally Accredited Y
Financial Aid   Y

Satellite Campus: N
International Students: Y
Number of International Students: NP

Program Uniqueness
NP

Faculty Research
NP

% faculty in professional counseling practice: NP

Program Accreditation

CACREP: Community Counseling; **CACREP:** School Counseling

Degree Programs
NP

Distance learning: N; 0% courses on-line: NP

Other Counseling Related Programs
NP

Faculty and Student Ethnicity
NP

Faculty
NP

Percent of faculty with NCC certification: NP

Other Credentials Held By Faculty Members
NP

Enrollment and Admission Requirements
NP

Graduation Requirements
NP

VA: Old Dominion University

Education Building, Room 110
Norfolk, VA 23529-0157
United States of America
http://education.odu.edu/chs/

Dean

Linda Irwin-DiVitis, Dean
Darden College of Education
218 Education Building
Norfolk, VA 23529
United States of America

Administrator

Danica Hays, Counseling Graduate Program Director
Education Building, Room 110
Old Dominion University
Norfolk, VA 23529-0157
United States of America
(757) 683-6692; fax: (757) 683-5756
dhays@odu.edu

CSI Chapter, Name   Y, Omega Delta
Regionally Accredited   Y
Financial Aid   Y

Satellite Campus: Y
International students: Y
Number of International students: 3

Program Uniqueness

Nationally-accredited by CACREP. Low faculty-to-student ratio. Awarded by the Association for Counselor Education and Supervision (ACES) the Outstanding Counselor Education Program in 2009.

Faculty Research

Group counseling and psychotherapy, narcissism, school counseling, multicultural counseling, supervision, qualitative methodology, assessment, clinical diagnosis, trauma, gender issues, multicultural and social advocacy issues in counselor preparation and mental health counseling, social and cultural diversity, constructivism, adult cognitive development, career decision-making, ethics, family systems, assessment, legal issues in counseling, integrating spirituality into counseling, caregiving for older adults and college counseling.

% faculty in professional counseling practice: NP

Program Accreditation

CACREP: College Counseling; **CACREP:** Community Counseling; **CACREP:** Counselor Education and Supervision; **CACREP:** Mental Health Counseling; **CACREP:** School Counseling

Degree Programs

Degree	Program	Contact
MEd	College Counseling	Danica Hays
MEd	Mental Health Counseling	Danica Hays
MEd	School Counseling	Danica Hays
EdS	Ed.S. in Counseling	Danica Hays
PhD	Counselor Education and Supervision	Danica Hays

Distance learning: Y; % courses on-line: NP

Other Counseling Related Programs

B.S. in HumanServices
M.S. in Psychology
Ph.D. in Psychology
Psy.D. in Clinical Psychology

Faculty and Student Ethnicity

Faculty	**Master's**	**Specialist**	**Doctoral**
African-American	African-American	African-American	African-American
Asian	Asian	Asian-American	Asian-American
Caucasian	Asian-American	Caucasian	Biracial
	Caucasian	Latino/Latina	Caucasian
	Latino/Latina	Multiracial	Pacific Islander
	Multiracial	Native American	
	Native American	Other	
	Pacific Islander		

Faculty

Name			Highest Degree	Rank	Time	Credentials State Lic.	NCC	Email
Brown	Nina		EdD	Full Professor		Y	Y	nbrown@odu.edu
Grothaus	Tim		PhD	Assistant Professor			Y	tgrothau@odu.edu
Hays	Danica	G	PhD	Associate Professor and Director of Counselor Education		Y	Y	dhays@odu.edu
Horton-Parker	Radha		PhD	Associate Professor			Y	rparker@odu.edu
McAuliffe	Garrett		EdD	Full Professor		Y	N	gmacaulif@odu.edu
Neukrug	Edward		EdD	Full Professor		Y	Y	eneukrug@odu.edu
Remley	Ted		PhD	Chair		Y	Y	tremley@odu.edu
Schwitzer	Alan		PhD	Associate Professor			N	aschwitz@odu.edu
Thompson	Suzan		PhD	Clinical Faculty		Y	N	skthomps@odu.edu

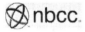 Percent of faculty with NCC certification: 66%   ncc

Other Credentials Held By Faculty Members: NP

Enrollment and Admission Requirements

Degree	Program	Gender F	M	Yearly Admit	Grad	GRE Total	MAT	Master	GPA	Work Exp	Letters	Interview
MEd	College Counseling	10	2	6	4			Y			3	N
MEd	Mental Health Counseling	56	14	35	35			Y			3	N
MEd	School Counseling	56	14	35	35			Y			3	N
EdS	Ed.S. in Counseling	4	1	2	1			Y			3	N
PhD	Counselor Education and Supervision	39	7	14	10			Y			3	Y

Graduation Requirements

Degree	Program	Academic Hours Sem	Qtr	Clock Hours Pract	Intern	Thesis	Examinations Comp	CPCE	Oral	Portfolio
MEd	College Counseling	48		100	600	N	Y	Y	N	N
MEd	Mental Health Counseling	60		100	600	N	Y	Y	N	N
MEd	School Counseling	48		100	600	N	Y	Y	N	Y
EdS	Ed.S. in Counseling	30				N	Y	N	N	N
PhD	Counselor Education and Supervision	60		100	600	Y	Y	N	Y	N

VA: University of Virginia

Counselor Education
Curry School
Bavaro Hall, Room 212D
417 Emmet Street South
Charlottesville, VA 22903
United States of America
http://curry.edschool.virginia.edu/counsed/

Dean

Robert Pianta, Professor and Dean
University of Virginia
Curry School of Education
P.O. Box 400261
Charlottesville, VA 22904-4261
United States of America

Administrator

Sandra I. Lopez-Baez
Associate Professor and Director of Counselor Education
University of Virginia
Curry School, Bavaro Hall
417 Emmet St. South, #218-G
Charlottesville, VA 22904-4269
United States of America
(434) 243-8716; fax: (434) 924-1433
slopez-baez@virginia.edu

CSI Chapter, Name   Y, Rho Beta
Regionally Accredited Y
Financial Aid   Y

Satellite Campus: N
International Students: N
Number of International Students: 0

Program Uniqueness

We admit full-time cohorts. Faculty members are active in leadership and service positions at the state, national and international level. In addition, the faculty as a whole infuses students' training experience with the application of concepts and skills to work with diverse clientele, including exploration of how issues of social justice and advocacy influence client work. Finally, there is a focus on intensive clinical supervision of students.

Faculty Research

Faculty members have a wide range of research and professional interests, including the following: ethical and legal issues in counseling, supervision and counseling education; multiculturalism and diversity; the role of spirituality and religion in counseling; advocacy and social justice issues related to counseling and supervision; counselor supervision research methods; white racial identity and consciousness; individual intervention techniques; biofeedback with Hispanic clients; counselor trainee qualities; training counselors in Latin America; human sexuality, feminist multicultural pedagogy; potential contributions of technology to counseling and counselor education; child and adolescent gender and career issues; collaborative training of school personnel; school counseling and consultation; supervision of supervision; psychoeducational assessment; counseling with children and adolescents; special populations in secondary schools and higher education; and student-athletes, wellness and career issues in the secondary school and college population.

25% faculty in professional counseling practice.

Program Accreditation

 CACREP: Counselor Education and Supervision; **CACREP:** School Counseling

CACREP

Degree Programs

Degree	Program	Contact
MEd	School Counseling	Marie L. Shoffner

Distance learning: N; % courses on-line: NP

Other Counseling Related Programs

Clinical Psychology

Faculty and Student Ethnicity

Faculty	Master's	Specialist	Doctoral
African-American	African-American		Multiracial
Latino/Latina	Latino/Latina		

Faculty

Name			Highest Degree	Rank	Time	State Lic.	NCC	Email
						Credentials		
Anderson	W.	P	PhD	Adjunct	<21	Y	N	wpa6n@virginia.edu
Doyle	Kevin		EdD	Adjunct	<21	Y	N	ksd3c@virginia.edu
Lopez-Baez	Sandra	I	PhD	Associate Professor		Y	Y	sll6f@virginia.edu
Shoffner	Marie	L	PhD	Associate Professor	>81	N	Y	mfs2@virginia.edu
Thomas	Antoinette	R	PhD	Associate Professor	41-60	N	N	art8u@virginia.edu
Williams, Jr.	Derick	J	PhD	Assistant Professor	>81	N	N	dw4pd@virginia.edu

 Percent of faculty with NCC certification: 33%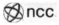

Other Credentials Held By Faculty Members: ACS, CCMHC, Licensed Psychologist, Licensed School Counselor, LMFT, LPC Supervisor, NCSC

Enrollment and Admission Requirements

Degree	Program	Gender F	M	Yearly Admit	Grad	GRE Total	MAT	Master	GPA	Work Exp	Letters	Interview
MEd	School Counseling	8	2	10	10	1000		Y	3		2	N

Graduation Requirements

Degree	Program	Academic Hours Sem	Qtr	Clock Hours Pract	Intern	Thesis	Comp	Examinations CPCE	Oral	Portfolio
MEd	School Counseling	49		100	600	N	Y	N	N	N

VA: Virginia Tech

308 East Eggleston Hall
Blacksburg, VA 24061-0302
United States of America
http://www.soe.vt.edu/counselored/

Dean

Sue Ott Rowlands
Dean of College of Liberal Arts and Human Sciences
Wallace Hall
Blacksburg, VA 24061
United States of America

Administrator

Elizabeth Creamer, Department Head
219 East Eggleston Hall
Blacksburg, VA 24061-0302
United States of America
(540) 231-5106; fax: (540) 231-7845
vmeadows@vt.edu

CSI Chapter, Name Y, Tau Eta Kappa and Tau Epsilon Kappa
Regionally Accredited Y
Financial Aid Y

Satellite Campus: Y
International Students: N
Number of International Students: 0

Program Uniqueness

Students are the first priority at both the master's and doctoral levels. Research and leadership are also highly valued. High tech instructional emphasis and a focus on intensive clinical supervision.

Faculty Research

Multicultural counseling competencies and counselor development, school counseling, clinical supervision, career development, play therapy, international counseling, and counselor development.

0% faculty in professional counseling practice.

Program Accreditation

CACREP: Community Counseling; **CACREP:** Counselor Education and Supervision; **CACREP:** School Counseling

Degree Programs

Degree	Program	Contact
M	Community Counseling	
M	School Counseling	
EdD	Counselor Education	
PhD	Counselor Education and Supervision	

Distance learning: Y; 5% courses on-line

Other Counseling Related Programs

Communications
Human Development
International Studies
Marriage and Family Therapists
Organizational Behaviorists
Psychology

Faculty and Student Ethnicity

Faculty	**Master's**	**Specialist**	**Doctoral**
African-American	African-American		African-American
Caucasian	Asian-American		Asian-American
	Caucasian		Caucasian
	Latino/Latina		Latino/Latina
	Multiracial		Multiracial

Faculty

Name		Highest Degree	Rank	Time	Credentials State Lic.	NCC	Email
Bodenhorn	Nancy	PhD	Associate Professor	>81		N	nanboden@vt.edu
Brott	Pamelia	PhD	Associate Professor	>81	N	N	pbrott@vt.edu
Day-Vines	Norma	PhD	Associate Professor	>81	N	N	ndayvine@vt.edu
Lambert	Simone	PhD	Assistant Professor	>81	Y	Y	slambert@vt.edu
Lawson	Gerard	PhD	Associate Professor	>81	Y	Y	glawson@vt.edu
Welfare	Laura	PhD	Assistant Professor	>81	Y	Y	welfare@vt.edu

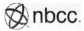   Percent of faculty with NCC certification: 50%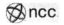

Other Credentials Held By Faculty Members: CAC, Certified School Counselor, LPC, LPC Supervisor

Enrollment and Admission Requirements

Degree	Program	Gender F	M	Yearly Admit	Grad	GRE Total	MAT	Master	GPA	Work Exp	Letters	Interview
M	Community Counseling	15	5	20	18	0			3		3	Y
M	School Counseling	15	5	20	18	0			3		3	Y
EdD	Counselor Education			0	0	0		Y	3		3	Y
PhD	Counselor Education and Supervision			7	6	0		Y	3	2	3	Y

Graduation Requirements

Degree	Program	Academic Hours Sem	Qtr	Clock Hours Pract	Intern	Thesis	Comp	Examinations CPCE	Oral	Portfolio
M	Community Counseling	51		100	600		Y	Y		
M	School Counseling	51		100	600		Y	Y		
EdD	Counselor Education	100			600	Y	Y		Y	
PhD	Counselor Education and Supervision	100		100	600	Y	Y		Y	

VT: Goddard College

123 Pitkin Road
Plainfield, VT 05667
United States of America
www.goddard.edu

Dean Lucinda Garthwaite, Academic Dean
123 Pitkin Road
Plainfield, VT 05667
United States of America

Administrator Steven James, Department Chair
10 Fairfield Drive
East Sandwich, MA 02537
United States of America
(978) 815-2480; fax: NP
steven.james@goddard.edu

CSI Chapter, Name N
Regionally Accredited Y
Financial Aid Y

Satellite Campus: Y
International Students: Y
Number of International Students: 4

Program Uniqueness

All courses are directed independent studies.

Faculty Research

NP

% faculty in professional counseling practice: NP

Degree Programs
NP

Distance learning: Y; 10% courses on-line

Other Counseling Related Programs
NP

Faculty and Student Ethnicity

Faculty	**Master's**	**Specialist**	**Doctoral**
African-American	African-American		
Caucasian	Asian-American		
Multiracial	Caucasian		
Native American	Latino/Latina		
	Multiracial		

Faculty
NP

Percent of faculty with NCC certification: NP

Other Credentials Held By Faculty Members
NP

Enrollment and Admission Requirements
NP

Graduation Requirements
NP

WA: Central Washington University

400 E. University Way
Department of Psychology, MS 7575
Ellensburg, WA 98926-7575
United States of America
http://www.cwu.edu/~counpsy/

Dean

Kirk Johnson, COTS Dean
College of the Sciences, MS 7519
400 E. University Way
Ellensburg, WA 98926
United States of America

Administrator

Robyn Brammer
Director of Mental Health and School Counseling
400 E. University Way
Ellensburg, WA 98926-7575
United States of America
(509) 963-2501; fax: (509) 963-2307

CSI Chapter, Name   Y, Chi Sigma Psi
Regionally Accredited Y
Financial Aid   Y

Satellite Campus: N
International Students: Y
Number of International Students: 20%

Program Uniqueness

Our programs continue to gain national and international recognition. We are only able to admit a small percentage of our applicants, but we are striving to admit students who add diversity. All of our faculty conduct research in multicultural and diversity issues, and students can expect to learn more about this as they move through the program. For example, Jeff Penick focuses on gerontology issues; Jennifer Cates addresses social justice and advocacy; Scott Schaefle works with Gear Up and other need-based groups; Robyn Brammer publishes on gender identity, ethnic immigration issues and spirituality; and Breyan Haizlip works on social class disparity, African American issues and sexuality. A strength of our CACREP-accredited programs is its unique balance between field experience and research. All of our students complete a research project or a thesis. We strongly advocate students to tie this research to work they are doing in their internship or with their faculty advisors, but students are free to do whatever interests them. Central also provides funding for students to present their research at national conferences.

Faculty Research

Counseling process research; self-efficacy; ADHD; developmental issues.

% faculty in professional counseling practice: NP

Program Accreditation

CACREP: Mental Health Counseling; **CACREP:** School Counseling

CACREP

Degree Programs

Degree	*Program*	*Contact*
MS	Mental Health Counseling	Robyn Brammer
MEd	School Counseling	Robyn Brammer

Distance learning: N; 0-3% courses on-line

Other Counseling Related Programs

Experimental Psychology / Applied Behavioral Analysis
School Psychology

Faculty and Student Ethnicity

Faculty	Master's	Specialist	Doctoral
African-American	African-American		
Caucasian	Asian		
Latino/Latina	Biracial		
	Caucasian		
	Latino/Latina		

Faculty

Name		Highest Degree	Rank	Time	Credentials State Lic.	NCC	Email
Brammer	Robyn	PhD	Associate Professor	41-60	Y	N	brammerr@cwu.edu
Haizlip	Breyan	PhD	Assistant Professor	61-80	Y	N	haizlipb@cwu.edu
Penick	Jeff	PhD	Associate Professor	61-80	Y	N	penickj@cwu.edu

Percent of faculty reported with NCC certification: 0%

Other Credentials Held By Faculty Members
NP

Enrollment and Admission Requirements

Degree	Program	Gender F	M	Yearly Admit	Grad	GRE Total	MAT	Master	GPA	Work Exp	Letters	Interview
MS	Mental Health Counseling	5	3	8	8	900		Y	3		3	N
MEd	School Counseling	3	2	5	4	900		Y	3			N

Graduation Requirements

Degree	Program	Academic Hours Sem	Qtr	Clock Hours Pract	Intern	Examinations Thesis	Comp	CPCE	Oral	Portfolio
MS	Mental Health Counseling	90		325	600	Y	Y	N	Y	Y
MEd	School Counseling	90		325	600	Y	Y	N	Y	Y

WA: Eastern Washington University

526 5th Street, MAR 213
Cheney, WA 99004
United States of America
www.ewu.edu

Dean
Alan Coelho
College of Education and Human Development

Administrator
Charlie Cleanthous, Director
526 5th Street, MAR 213
Cheney, WA 99004
United States of America
(509) 359-2816; fax: (509) 359-4366
ccleanthous@ewu.edu

CSI Chapter, Name Y, Epsilon Alpha Psi Chapter
Regionally Accredited Y
Financial Aid Y

Satellite Campus: Y
International Students: N
Number of International Students: 0

Program Uniqueness

CACREP accredited programs in school counseling and mental health counseling.

Faculty Research

Career, bilingual/multicultural, narrative and family counseling.

% faculty in professional counseling practice: NP

Program Accreditation

CACREP: Mental Health Counseling; **CACREP:** School Counseling

Degree Programs

Degree	Program	Contact
M	Mental Health Counseling	Alan Basham, M.A.
M	School Counseling	Marty Slyter, Ph.D.

Distance learning: N; 0% courses on-line

Other Counseling Related Programs
NP

Faculty and Student Ethnicity

Faculty	Master's	Specialist	Doctoral
African-American			
Caucasian			
Latino/Latina			
Native American			

Faculty

Name		Highest Degree	Rank	Time	Credentials State Lic.	NCC	Email
Engbresson	Ken					N	
Leverett	Sarah					N	

Percent of faculty with NCC certification: 0%

Other Credentials Held by Faculty Members
NP

Enrollment and Admission Requirements

Degree	Program	Gender F	M	Yearly Admit	Grad	GRE Total	MAT	Master	GPA	Work Exp	Letters	Interview
M	Mental Health Counseling			12	12			Y			2	Y
M	School Counseling			12	12							

Graduation Requirements

Degree	Program	Academic Hours Sem	Qtr	Clock Hours Pract	Intern	Thesis	Comp	Examinations CPCE	Oral	Portfolio
M	Mental Health Counseling									
M	School Counseling									

WA: Seattle Pacific University

School of Education
Seattle Pacific University
3307 3rd Ave. West
Seattle, WA 98119-1997
United States of America
http://sites.google.com/site/spucounseloreducation/

Dean

Rick Eigenbrood
Seattle Pacific University
School of Education
3307 3rd Ave. West
Seattle, WA 98119-1997
United States of America

Administrator

Cher Edwards
Seattle Pacific University
School of Education
3307 3rd Ave. West
Seattle, WA 98119-1997
United States of America
(206) 281-2286; fax: (206) 281-2756
edwards@spu.edu

CSI Chapter, Name   NP
Regionally Accredited Y
Financial Aid   Y

Satellite Campus: N
International Students: Y
Number of International Students: 2

Program Uniqueness

Comprehensive school programs, advocacy, family work, multicultural counseling, spirituality, ethics and values.

Faculty Research

Comprehensive school counseling, at risk, multicultural counseling, social justice, family issues, psychoeducational assessment, and program evaluation.

50% faculty in professional counseling practice.

Degree Programs

Degree	Program	Contact
M	School Counseling	Cher Edwards
PhD	Counselor Education	Cher Edwards
EdD	School Counseling	Cher Edwards

Distance learning: N; 10% courses on-line

Other Counseling Related Programs

MFT: Marriage and Family Therapy
Ph.D. Clinical Psychology
Ph.D. Organizational Psychology

Faculty and Student Ethnicity

Faculty	Master's	Specialist	Doctoral
Asian	African-American		Biracial
Caucasian	Asian		Caucasian
	Asian-American		Other
	Biracial		Pacific Islander
	Caucasian		
	Latino/Latina		
	Multiracial		
	Native American		

Faculty

Name			Highest Degree	Rank	Time	Credentials State Lic.	NCC	Email
Edwards	Cher		PhD	Associate Professor and Chair		Y	N	edwards@spu.edu
Hyun	June	A	PhD	Assistant Professor	<21	N	N	jhyun@spu.edu
Sink	Christopher		PhD	Full Professor	<21	Y	Y	csink@spu.edu

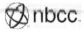 Percent of faculty with NCC certification: 33%

Other Credentials Held By Faculty Members: LMHP, LPC Supervisor

Enrollment and Admission Requirements

Degree	Program	Gender F	M	Yearly Admit	Grad	GRE Total	MAT	Master	GPA	Work Exp	Letters	Interview
M	School Counseling	18	2	20	18	1000	400	Y	3.2	1	2	Y
PhD	Counselor Education	2	1	3	1	1200		Y		2	3	Y
EdD	School Counseling	2	1	3							4	Y

Graduation Requirements

Degree	Program	Academic Hours Sem	Qtr	Clock Hours Pract	Intern	Thesis	Comp	Examinations CPCE	Oral	Portfolio
M	School Counseling		72	100	600	N	Y	N	N	Y
PhD	Counselor Education									
EdD	School Counseling		90	100	600	Y	Y			Y

WA: University of Puget Sound

1500 N. Warner CMB#1051
Tacoma, WA 98416-1051
United States of America
http://www.pugetsound.edu/academics/departments-and-
programs/graduate/school-of-education/

Dean   John Woodward, Dean of the School of Education
1500 N. Warner Street CMB#1051
Tacoma, WA 98416-1051
United States of America

Administrator   Anna Coy, Administrative Assistant
1500 N. Warner CMB#1051
Tacoma, WA 98416-1051
United States of America
(253) 879-3375; fax: (253) 879-3926

CSI Chapter, Name   NP
Regionally Accredited   Y
Financial Aid   Y

Satellite Campus: N
International Students: N
Number of International Students: 0

Program Uniqueness

Validity of admissions criteria to screen candidates for graduate study. Administrators' perceptions of school counselors' roles.

Faculty Research

Students study a wide range of counseling theories and learn to apply them in a variety of contexts.

50% faculty in professional counseling practice.

Degree Programs

Degree	Program	Contact
M	Mental Health Counseling	Grace Kirchner
M	School Counseling	Grace Kirchner

Distance learning: N; 0% courses on-line

Other Counseling Related Programs

Occupational Therapy
Physical Therapy
Psychology

Faculty and Student Ethnicity

Faculty	Master's	Specialist	Doctoral
Caucasian	African-American		
	Asian-American		
	Caucasian		
	Latino/Latina		
	Pacific Islander		

Faculty

Name			Highest Degree	Rank	Time	Credentials State Lic.	NCC	Email
Gast	Joan	E	MEd	Instructor	>81	Y	N	bgast@ups.edu
Kirchner	Grace	L	PhD	Full Professor	>81		N	kirchner@ups.edu
Smith	Jerry		MEd	Adjunct	<21	Y	N	smithjf@comcast.net
Woodward	John		PhD	Full Professor	<21		N	woodward@ups.edu

Percent of faculty with NCC certification: 0%

Other Credentials Held By Faculty Members: NP

Enrollment and Admission Requirements

Degree	Program	Gender F	M	Yearly Admit	Grad	GRE Total	MAT	Master	GPA	Work Exp	Letters	Interview
M	Mental Health Counseling	5	1	6	6	1500			3		2	Y
M	School Counseling	5	1	6	6	1500			3		2	Y

Graduation Requirements

Degree	Program	Academic Hours Sem	Qtr	Clock Hours Pract	Intern	Thesis	Examinations Comp	CPCE	Oral	Portfolio
M	Mental Health Counseling	48		32	400		Y		Y	
M	School Counseling	48		32	400		Y		Y	

WA: Western Washington University

516 High Street
Bellingham, WA 98226-9172
United States of America
www.ac.wwu.edu/~psych/

Dean Brent Carbajal

Administrator Dale L. Dinnel, Chairperson
516 High Street
Bellingham, WA 98226-9172
United States of America
(360) 650-3515; fax: (360) 650-7305

CSI Chapter, Name NP
Regionally Accredited Y
Financial Aid Y

Satellite Campus: N
International Students: Y
Number of International Students: 1

Program Uniqueness

Highly selective, small, full-time programs in school and mental health counseling.

Faculty Research

Peer helping programs, women and anger expression, youth substance use, domestic violence, multicultural counseling, psychological resilience in children, couple relationship quality, children and parental conflict.

20% faculty in professional counseling practice.

Program Accreditation

CACREP: Mental Health Counseling; **CACREP:** School Counseling

Degree Programs

Degree	Program	Contact
M	Mental Health Counseling	Christina Byrne
M	School Counseling	Diana Gruman

Distance learning: N; 0% courses on-line

Other Counseling Related Programs
NP

Faculty and Student Ethnicity

Faculty	Master's	Specialist	Doctoral
Asian	African-American		
Caucasian	Asian-American		
	Caucasian		
	Native American		

Faculty

Name			Highest Degree	Rank	Time	Credentials State Lic.	NCC	Email
Bedi	Robinder		PhD	Assistant Professor	61-80	N	N	Rob.Bedi@wwu.edu
Byrne	Christina		PhD	Associate Professor	61-80	N	N	Christina.Byrne@wwu.edu
DuRocher-Schudlich	Tina		PhD	Assistant Professor	61-80	N	N	Tina.Schudlich@wwu.edu
Forgays	Deborah	K	PhD	Full Professor	61-80	N	N	Deborah.Forgays@wwu.edu
Graham	Jim		PhD	Associate Professor	41-60	N	N	James.Graham@wwu.edu
Gruman	Diana		PhD	Associate Professor	61-80	N	Y	Diana.Gruman@wwu.edu
Lewis	Arleen	C	PhD	Full Professor	>81	Y	N	Arleen.Lewis@wwu.edu

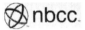 Percent of faculty with NCC certification: 14%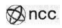

Other Credentials Held By Faculty Members: Certified School Counselor, Licensed Psychologist

Enrollment and Admission Requirements

Degree	Program	Gender F	M	Yearly Admit	Grad	Total	GRE Total	MAT	Master	GPA	Work Exp	Letters	Interview
M	Mental Health Counseling	4	2	6	6				Y	3		3	Y
M	School Counseling	4	2	6	6				Y	3		3	Y

Graduation Requirements

Degree	Program	Academic Hours Sem	Qtr	Clock Hours Pract	Intern	Thesis	Comp	Examinations CPCE	Oral	Portfolio
M	Mental Health Counseling		91	300	700	N	Y			
M	School Counseling		83	100	600	N	Y			

WI: Marquette University

College of Education
561 N. 15th Street
Department of Counselor Education and Counseling Psychology
Milwaukee, WI 53233
United States of America
http://www.marquette.edu/education/grad/index.shtml

Dean   William Henk
College of Education
561 N. 15th Street
Milwaukee, WI 53233
United States of America

Administrator   Alan Burkard, Chair
Marquette University
School of Education
561 N. 15th Street
Milwaukee, WI 53233
United States of America
(414) 288-5790; fax: (414) 288-6100
alan.burkard@marquette.edu

CSI Chapter, Name   N
Regionally Accredited Y
Financial Aid   Y

Satellite Campus: N
International Students: N
Number of International Students: 0

Program Uniqueness

Our master's program in counseling includes a variety of courses, practicum, internship and other training experiences which offer comprehensive preparation for the practice as a professional counselor. Training in counseling skills begins in the first semester, practicum experiences start in the first year and formalized internships begin in the second year. Full-time students complete the program in two years. We offer the following specializations: Community Counseling - Prepares students for positions in health care organizations, community mental health agencies, private practice and college counseling centers. Child and Adolescent Counseling - Within the Community Counseling program, this specialization offers additional training specific to providing counseling services to children and adolescents and their families. Addiction Counseling - Our Addiction Counseling Track is one of the specialty areas within the Community Counseling Program and is geared toward working with adults with substance abuse disorders. School Counseling - Prepares students to work as school counselors in both primary and secondary schools, providing mental health and academic services; meets DPI licensure requirements.

Faculty Research

All of the full-time faculty are engaged in a variety of research projects with which students may become involved. Alan Burkard, Ph.D., research interests: supervision, multicultural issues, school counseling. Lisa Edwards, Ph.D., research interests: multicultural counseling strengths and positive functioning, Latino/a Psychology, biracial/multiracial identity. Todd C. Campbell, Ph.D., research interests: addiction and mental health, motivational interviewing, one treatment processes assessment. Sarah Knox, Ph.D., research interests: therapy relationship, qualitative research training and supervision, mental health of clergy. Tim Melchert, Ph.D., research interests: theories of counseling and psychotherapy, research methods, clinical practicum, professional ethics and legal issues. Bob Fox, Ph.D., research interests: in-home child management therapy, child psychopathology, developmental disabilities. Rebecca Bardwell, Ph.D., research interests: organizational change and program evaluation, ethical and legal issues in education, motivation, affective education, and positive psychology.

14% faculty in professional counseling practice.

Degree Programs

Degree	Program	Contact
MA	Community Counseling	Alan Burkard
MA	School Counseling	Alan Burkard

Distance learning: N; 0% courses on-line

Other Counseling Related Programs
NP

Faculty and Student Ethnicity

Faculty	Master's	Specialist	Doctoral
Caucasian	African-American		
Latino/Latina	Caucasian		
	Latino/Latina		

Faculty

Name		Highest Degree	Rank	Time	Credentials State Lic.	NCC	Email
Bardwell	Rebecca	PhD	Associate Professor	61-80	N	N	rebecca.bardwell@mu.edu
Burkard	Alan	PhD	Associate Professor and Chair	22-40	N	N	alan.burkard@mu.edu
Campbell	Todd	PhD	Associate Professor	61-80	N	N	todd.campbell@mu.edu
Edwards	Lisa	PhD	Assistant Professor	61-80	N	N	lisa.edwards@mu.edu
Fox	Robert	PhD	Full Professor	41-60	N	Y	robert.fox@marquette.edu
Knox	Sarah	PhD	Associate Professor	41-60	N	N	sarah.knox@mu.edu
Melchert	Tim	PhD	Associate Professor	41-60	N	Y	timothy.melchert@mu.edu

   Percent of faculty with NCC certification: 29%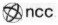

Other Credentials Held By Faculty Members: Licensed Psychologist

Enrollment and Admission Requirements

Degree	Program	Gender F	M	Yearly Admit	Grad	GRE Total	MAT	Master	GPA	Work Exp	Letters	Interview
MA	Community Counseling	25	5	30	28			Y		0	3	Y
MA	School Counseling	9	1	10	0			Y		0	3	Y

Graduation Requirements

Degree	Program	Academic Hours Sem	Qtr	Clock Hours Pract	Intern	Thesis	Examinations Comp	CPCE	Oral	Portfolio
MA	Community Counseling	48		100	600	N	Y	Y	N	Y
MA	School Counseling	48		100	600	N	Y	N	N	Y

WI: University of Wisconsin-Whitewater

6035 Winther Hall
Whitewater, WI 53190-0296
United States of America
http://academics.uww.edu/counseled/

Dean
Katy Heyning
College of Education

Administrator
Donald Norman, Ph.D.
Associate Professor and Chairperson
6035 Winther Hall
UW-Whitewater
Whitewater, WI 53190-0296
United States of America
(262) 472-5426; fax: (262) 472-2841
counslred@mail.uww.edu

CSI Chapter, Name   Y, Zeta Omicron Omega
Regionally Accredited Y
Financial Aid   Y

Satellite Campus: N
International Students: Y
Number of International Students: 2

Program Uniqueness

It is a 48-credit program with three major emphases: community, higher education, and school. It is also a CACREP-accredited program that emphasizes diversity/multiculturalism in its curriculum.

Faculty Research: NP

% faculty in professional counseling practice: NP

Program Accreditation

CACREP: College Counseling; **CACREP:** Community Counseling; **CACREP:** School Counseling; **CACREP:** Student Affairs

Degree Programs

Degree	Program	Contact
M	Community Counseling	
M	School Counseling	
M	Student Affairs	

Distance learning: N; 10% courses on-line

Other Counseling Related Programs
NP

Faculty and Student Ethnicity

Faculty	**Master's**	**Specialist**	**Doctoral**
African-American	African-American		
Caucasian	Asian-American		
	Caucasian		
	Latino/Latina		

Faculty

Name		Highest Degree	Rank	Time	Credentials State Lic.	NCC	Email
Curtis	Gregg	PhD	Assistant Professor	>81	N	N	curtisg@uww.edu
Downs	Joni	PhD	Assistant Professor	>81	N	N	downsj@uww.edu
Norman	Donald	PhD	Associate Professor and Chair		Y	N	normand@mail.uww.edu
O'Beirne	Brenda	PhD	Associate Professor	>81		N	obeirneb@mail.uww.edu
Okocha	Aneneosa	PhD	Full Professor	>81		Y	okochaa@mail.uww.edu
Van Doren	David	EdD	Associate Professor		Y	Y	vandored@mail.uww.edu

 Percent of faculty with NCC certification: 33%

Other Credentials Held By Faculty Members: AAMFT Approved Supervisor, CCMHC, Licensed Psychologist, LPC, MAC

Enrollment and Admission Requirements

Degree	*Program*	*Gender* F M	*Yearly* Admit Grad	GRE Total	MAT	Master	GPA	Work Exp	Letters	Interview
M	Community Counseling		27 23				2.75		2	Y
M	School Counseling		23 16				2.75		2	Y
M	Student Affairs		5 3				2.75		2	Y

Graduation Requirements

Degree	*Program*	*Academic Hours* Sem Qtr	*Clock Hours* Pract Intern	Thesis	Comp	*Examinations* CPCE	Oral	Portfolio
M	Community Counseling	48	100 640					
M	School Counseling	48	100 640					
M	Student Affairs	48	100 640					

Data on Each Department Outside the United States

AUSTRALIA: Australian College of Applied Psychology

Level 5, 11 York St.
Sydney NSW 2206
Australia
acap.edu.au

Dean   Dr. Ed Green
Level 5, 11 York St.
Sydney NSW 2206
Australia

Administrator   NP

Regionally Accredited NP
Financial Aid   NP

Program Uniqueness

At ACAP, we believe that the only way for one to learn how to build relationships and communicate effectively with people is to do just that. So we have designed an approach to learning that allows students to put the theory they learn straight into practice. With campuses in Sydney, Brisbane and Melbourne, and the majority of our courses offered by flexible delivery, we give our students (depending on the course they select) the option to choose where and how they want to study.

Faculty Research
NP

% faculty in professional counseling practice: NP

Degree Programs

Degree	*Program*	*Contact*
Bachelor of Applied Social Science	Counselling	
Graduate Diploma of Counselling	Counselling	
Master of Applied Social Science		

Distance learning: NP; NP % courses on-line

Faculty
NP

Enrollment and Admission Requirements

Degree	Program	Enrollment and Admission Requirement
Bachelor of Applied Social Science	Counselling	Please refer to the ACAP website for details.
Graduate Diploma of Counselling Master of Applied Social Science	Counselling	Please refer to the ACAP website, www.acap.edu.au, for details.

Graduation Requirements

Degree	Program	Duration	Practicum	Internship	Thesis/ Dissertation	Comp	Oral	Portfolio
Bachelor of Applied Social Science	Counselling	3		Y	N	N	N	N

The Bachelor of Applied Social Science (Counselling) is ideal if a student is interested in working as a counsellor in a variety of areas of specialisation or in a counselling related profession. Completing this course will provide the student with practical counselling skills and a firm understanding of the social and environmental contexts that impact an individual in today's society. With over 26 years of experience in teaching counselling, our small class sizes and hands-on approach to learning vital communication, counselling, behavior, and psychology skills will give the student an advantage in this growing field.

Degree	Program	Duration	Practicum	Internship	Thesis/ Dissertation	Comp	Oral	Portfolio
Grdauate Diploma of Counselling	Counselling	2		Y	N	N	N	N
Master of Applied Social Science		2		N		N	N	N

Counselling others to overcome problems in their lives is a rewarding and challenging career. If a student already has a degree in any discipline and would like to gain a qualification toward becoming a counsellor in just two years, the Graduate Diploma of Counselling will give him or her the practical skills needed. Students will learn to apply the theoretical and ethical foundations of counselling to a range of practical situations while also learning about conflict management, mental health issues and developmental psychology. If a student chooses to study solely by flexible delivery, he or she will need to attend three weeks of on-campus workshops to ensure getting the most from this interactive learning environment and to meet PACFA's training standards. Students may also choose to take this study further with advanced standing to the Master of Applied Social Science (Counselling) at ACAP. Working as a counsellor is an enriching experience, and this Master's program allows students to continue to develop specialised skills, apply the latest research developments to practical cases and sharpen the understanding of the latest issues. This two-year program is designed for those already working as counsellors and combines a high level of academic rigour with ACAP's uniquely practical approach to learning.

BULGARIA: Sofia University

St. Kliment Ohridski
15, Tzar Osvoboditel Str., Room 56
Sofia 1504
Bulgaria

Dean
Ivaylo Tepavicharov, Ph.D., Associate Professor
15, Tzar Osvoboditel Str., Room 22
Sofia 1504
Bulgaria

Administrator
Silvia Tsvetanska, Ph.D., Associate Professor
15, Tzar Osvoboditel Str., Room 22
Sofia 1504
Bulgaria
telephone: +35929894563; fax: +359 28464085
silviatzvetanska@abv.bg

Regionally Accredited NP
Financial Aid NP

Program Uniqueness
NP

Faculty Research
NP

% faculty in professional counseling practice: NP

Degree Programs

Degree	*Program*	*Contact*
Master	Professional Qualification	

Distance learning: N; 0% courses on-line

Faculty
NP

Enrollment and Admission Requirements

Degree	Program	*Enrollment and Admission Requirement*
Master's	Professional Qualification	

Graduation Requirements

Degree	Program	Duration	Practicum	Internship	Thesis/ Dissertation	Comp	Oral	Portfolio
Master	Professional Qualification	1 year		Y	N	Y	Y	Y

CANADA: University of British Columbia

Department of Educational and Counselling Psychology,
and Special Education
University of British Columbia Faculty of Education
2125 Main Mall
Vancouver, B.C. V6T 1Z4
Canada

Dean   NP

Administrator   NP

Regionally Accredited NP
Financial Aid   NP

Program Uniqueness
NP

Faculty Research
NP

% faculty in professional counseling practice: NP

Degree Programs
NP

Distance learning: NP; NP % courses on-line

Faculty
NP

Enrollment and Admission Requirements
NP

Graduation Requirements
NP

GERMANY: Fachhochschule Frankfurt am Main - University of Applied Sciences

Nibelungenplatz 1
Frankfurt am Main, Hessia 60318
Germany

Dean   NP

Administrator   NP

Regionally Accredited NP
Financial Aid   NP

Program Uniqueness
NP

Faculty Research
NP

% faculty in professional counseling practice: NP

Degree Programs
NP

Distance learning: NP; NP % courses on-line

Faculty
NP

Enrollment and Admission Requirements
NP

Graduation Requirements
NP

GREECE: Institute of Counselling and Psychological Studies (ICPS)

56a Filikon Street Ag. Antonios - Peristeri
Athens 121 31
Greece

Dean   Ms. Polly Iossifides
56a Filikon Street
Ag. Antonios - Peristeri
Athens 121 31
Greece

Administrator   Ms. Polly Lossifides
56a Filikon Street
Ag. Antonios - Peristeri
Athens, 121 31
Greece
telephone: +30 210 64 56 564; fax: +30 210 64 54 982
p.iossifides@icps.edu.gr

Regionally Accredited NP
Financial Aid   NP

Program Uniqueness
NP

Faculty Research
NP

% faculty in professional counseling practice: NP

Degree Programs

Degree	*Program*	*Contact*
	Counselling Skills	Admissions Office
Master of Science (M.Sc.)	Person-Centred Counselling	Admissions Office
Postgraduate Certificate (Pg.Cert)	Person-Centred Counselling	Admissions Office
Postgraduate Diploma (Pg.Dip.)	Person-Centred Counselling	Admissions Office

Distance learning: NP; NP % courses on-line

Faculty
NP

Enrollment and Admission Requirements

Degree	Program	Enrollment and Admission Requirement
	Counselling Skills	
Master of Science (M.Sc.)	M.Sc. in Person-Centered Counselling	Successful completion of the Postgraduate Diploma in Person-Centered Counselling
Postgraduate Certificate (Pg.Cert)	Person-Centered Counselling	
Postgraduate Diploma (Pg.Dip.)	Person-Centered Counselling	Successful completion of the Postgraduate Certificate in Person-Centered Counselling

Graduation Requirements

Degree	Program	Duration	Practicum	Internship	Thesis/ Dissertation	Comp	Oral	Portfolio
	Counselling Skills	1 year		N	N	N	Y	Y
Master of Science (M.Sc.)	M.Sc. in Person-Centred Counselling	1 year		N	Y	N	Y	Y
Postgraduate Certificate (Pg Cert)	Person-Centred Counselling	2 years		N	N	N	Y	Y
Postgraduate Diploma (Pg.Dip.)	Person-Centred Counselling	1 year		N	N	N	Y	Y

A Postgraduate Certificate program leading to the award of Master of Science in Person-Centred Counselling of the University of Strathclyde (UK).
A Postgraduate Certificate program leading to the award of Postgraduate Certificate in Person-Centered Counselling of the University of Strathclyde (UK).
A Postgraduate Certificate program leading to the award of Postgraduate Diploma in Person-Centered Counselling of the University of Strathclyde (UK).

GREECE: The American College of Greece, DEREE

6 Gravias Street
Athens 15342 Aghia Paraskevi
Greece
http://www.acg.edu/ms-applied-psychology

Dean   Dr. Todd Fritch
Vice President of Academic Affairs
and Dean of Graduate and Professional Studies
6 Gravias Street
Athens 15342 Aghia Paraskevi
Greece

Administrator   Dr. Fotini-Sonia Apergi
Coordinator, M.S. in Applied Psychology
6 Gravias School
Athens 15342 Aghia Paraskevi
Greece
telephone: 30 210 6009800; fax: NP
tapergi@acg.edu

Regionally Accredited NP
Financial Aid   NP

Program Uniqueness

The M.S. in Applied Psychology is a two-year program designed for students who wish to explore links and establish bridges between theory, research and practice related to counseling and development. The core aim of the M.S. in Applied Psychology is to prepare students to become academically knowledgeable, competent and ethically responsible professionals. The program emphasizes evidence-based practice (including the development of applied counseling skills and behavioral analytic techniques), the use of quantitative and qualitative methods, and program evaluation. Students are trained to conduct assessment of clients and program needs, and to design and implement interventions that integrate therapeutic and developmental requirements.

The program has a number of distinct features: 1) Theoretical Integration: Integrative in theoretical orientation, the program provides an introduction and exposure to major theoretical approaches to counseling and psychotherapy. 2) Theory to Practice: Coursework is designed to provide a sequential progression from knowledge base to skill development to application through the incorporation of applied components in class and practicum experience in the field. 3) Specializations: Students can choose between two different areas that allow for specialization in adult and child/adolescent populations. At the same time, students have freedom of choice with respect to the experience gained through the different practica placements.
- Counseling Psychology: This is oriented toward people experiencing and expressing a wide range of pathology and aims at helping them to alleviate distress and maladjustment, resolve crises and increase their ability to live functional lives. It encompasses all age groups, with sensitivity to cultural differences and an emphasis on the strengths and adaptive strategies of an individual across his or her life span.
- Applied Developmental Psychology: This recognizes the importance of a developmental approach to understanding both normal and atypical human behavior. It focuses on the applications of knowledge and research regarding human development. Developmental theory and research are used to generate interventions that can enhance functioning and promote positive developmental outcomes in individuals, families and communities.
- Scientist-Practitioner Approach: The program is based on the scientist practitioner model and the belief that a competent practitioner must have both a broad knowledge of scientific and theoretical principles and the ability to apply that knowledge to specific situations with sensitivity to client needs and diversity issues.

Faculty Research
NP

80% faculty in professional counseling practice.

Degree Programs

Degree	Program	Contact
Graduate Certificate	Graduate Certificate in Applied Behavioral Analysis (ABA)	Dr. Fotini-Sonia Apergi
MS	MS in Applied Psychology	Dr. Fotini-Sonia Apergi

Distance learning: N; 0% courses on-line

Faculty

Name		Highest Degree	Rank	Email
Apergi	Fotini-Sonia	Psy.D.	Professor I, Graduate Faculty, Program Coordinator	tapergi@acg.edu
Janikian	Mari	Ph.D.	Professor I, Graduate Faculty	mjanikian@acg.edu
Pelios	Lilian	Ph.D.	Adjunct Professor, Graduate Faculty	lpelios@acg.edu
Takis	Nikos	Ph.D.	Professor I, Graduate Faculty	ntakis@acg.edu

Enrollment and Admission Requirements

Degree	Program	Enrollment and Admission Requirement
Graduate Certificate	Graduate Certificate in Applied Behavioral Analysis (ABA)	1. Completed application form (including essays on separate sheets). 2. Passport size photograph. 3. Official college or university transcript of undergraduate degree studies from an accredited institution. 4.Official college or university transcript of graduate degree studies from an accredited institution (if applicable). 5. Evidence of proficiency in English. 6. A certified copy of an identification card (for Greek citizens) or of a valid passport (for non-Greeks). Candidates are also required to attend an interview with representatives of the Graduate Studies Committee. The Graduate Studies Committee will review an application upon submission of all required documentation to the Office of Admissions. There is no application fee. Evidence of Proficiency in English: All candidates must provide evidence of proficiency in the English language by submitting one of the following: 1.TOEFL. 2.Cambridge or Michigan Proficiency Certificate. 3. GCE. 4. International Baccalaureate Certificate or Diploma. 5. International English Language Testing System (IELTS). Note: DEREE College graduates and graduates from other accredited English language institutions are not required to submit evidence of proficiency in the English language. Applicants presenting a TOEFL score should arrange to have the test results sent directly to the Office of Admissions by the Educational Testing Service (ETS). The College's Institution Code Number is 0925. TOEFL scores are valid for two years. Conditional Admission: Applicants who do not meet the minimum criteria may be admitted to the program on conditional status if the Graduate Studies Committee perceives other strengths in their application (e.g., strong research or relevant work experience, or other outstanding achievements during the applicants' undergraduate experience). In such cases, applicants will be expected to complete the requirements of the conditional admission within a specified period of time. Failure to complete these requirements will result in notification of dismissal by the Dean of the Graduate School. Students who have potential but lack the necessary prerequisites may be offered conditional admission and will be required to successfully complete preparatory courses prior to being fully admitted. Interview: Once a complete application package has been submitted, the Office of Admissions will contact the applicant to arrange an on-campus interview with representatives of the Graduate Studies Committee.

MS	MS in Applied Psychology

The following are required of all Graduate School applicants: 1.Completed application form (including essays on separate sheets). 2. Passport size photograph. 3. Two recommendation letters (at least one from an academic source and one from an employer, the latter highly recommended for MBA candidates). 4. Official college or university transcript of undergraduate degree studies from an accredited institution. 5. Official college or university transcript of graduate degree studies from an accredited institution (if applicable). 6. Evidence of proficiency in English. 7. A certified copy of an identification card for Greek citizens or of a valid passport for non-Greek Candidates are also required to attend an interview with the respective Graduate Program Coordinator. The Graduate Program Coordinators will review an application upon submission of all required documentation to the Office of Admissions. There is no application fee. Transfer applicants should refer to the section entitled "Transfer Students." Non-degree applicants should refer to the section entitled "Degree and Non-Degree Students." Evidence of Proficiency in English: All candidates must provide evidence of proficiency in the English language by submitting one of the following: 1.TOEFL. 2.Cambridge, Michigan Proficiency Certificate or Michigan State University Certificate. 3. GCE. 4. International Baccalaureate Certificate or Diploma. 5. International English Language Testing System (IELTS). Note: DEREE College graduates and graduates from other accredited English language institutions are not required to submit evidence of proficiency in the English language. Applicants presenting a TOEFL score should arrange to have the test results sent directly to the Office of Admissions by the Educational Testing Service (ETS). The College's Institution Code Number is 0925. TOEFL scores are valid for two years. Letters of Recommendation: Each applicant for admission must submit two letters of recommendation. At least one of the references must be from an academic source. One letter from an employer is highly recommended for MBA candidates. A letter from a family member or a friend is not admissible. Conditional Admission: Applicants who do not meet the minimum criteria may be admitted to the program on conditional status if the Graduate Program Coordinator perceives other strengths in the application (e.g., strong research or relevant work experience, or other outstanding achievements during the applicant's undergraduate experience). In such cases, applicants will be expected to complete the requirements of the conditional admission within a specified period of time. Failure to complete these requirements will result in notification of dismissal by the Dean of the Graduate School. Students who have potential but lack the necessary prerequisites may be offered conditional admission and will be required to successfully complete preparatory courses prior to being fully admitted. Interview: Once a complete application package has been submitted, the Office of Admissions will contact the applicant to arrange an on-campus interview with the respective Graduate Program Coordinator. Prerequisite courses: All applicants, regardless of specialization, should have completed at least: •2 introductory courses in psychology •1 course in statistics •1 course in research methods in psychology •1 course in developmental psychology •1 course in theories of personality •1 course in psychopathology. Those wishing to follow the graduate program in Applied Developmental Psychology should have also completed one additional course in Developmental Psychology.

Graduation Requirements

Degree	Program	Duration	Practicum	Internship	Thesis/ Dissertation	Comp	Oral	Portfolio
Graduate Certificate	Graduate Certificate in Applied Behavioral Analysis (ABA)	1 year	Y	N	N	N		

The Graduate Certificate (GC) in ABA is designed for professionals who are at various stages in their professional development. Specifically: •Psychology practitioners with or without a graduate degree who wish to extend their expertise in the area of ABA and Autism. •Persons who have recently completed their undergraduate studies in psychology and wish to acquire expertise in the area of behavior analysis and autism but do not have the time or money to pursue a graduate degree. •Psychologists with a master's degree, who wish to extend their expertise in ABA and autism. Approved applicants for the GC in ABA must complete a total of 17 credit hours (14 credits of course work hours and 3 credits in practicum experience). The GC is designed so that it can be completed within an academic year.

MS	MS in Applied Psychology	2 years		Y	Y			

The program is based on the scientist/practitioner model. That model is grounded in the belief that a competent practitioner must have both a broad knowledge of the scientific and theoretical principles and the ability to apply that knowledge to specific situations with sensitivity to diversity issues. Courses are designed so that they progress sequentially from knowledge base to skill development to application. Students are given the opportunity to explore the most current research in a chosen area of study, which provides excellent preparation for those wishing to continue their studies and pursue a doctoral degree. Additionally, the scientific emphasis of the program prepares students to critically examine the practice of psychology. The program consists of a set of core courses and two specializations in Applied Psychology: Counseling Psychology and Applied Developmental Psychology. Integrative in orientation, the M.S. in Applied Psychology provides a basic introduction to major theoretical approaches to counseling and psychotherapy. The counseling and applied developmental tracks allow a specialization in both adult and child populations, while the program offers freedom of choice with respect to the experience students gain through the different practica placements. This is a two-year program that students must complete successfully with a minimum of 50 credits, which includes a research thesis and practicum. Courses are offered in the afternoon hours and are supplemented by experiential workshops and a colloquia series. All students are expected to complete 40 hours of personal therapy with a qualified professional while enrolled in the M.S. in Applied Psychology program, regardless of previous personal therapy experience.

GREECE: University of Indianapolis Athens Campus

	Ipitou 9
	Athens 10557
	Greece

Dean Chancellor Mr. V. J. Botopoulos
Ipitou 9
Athens 10557
Greece

Administrator Dr. Anastasia P. Rush, Chair
Ipitou 9
Athens 10557
Greece
telephone: +30 210 3237077; fax: +30 210 3248502
rusha@uindy.gr

Regionally Accredited NP
Financial Aid NP

Program Uniqueness

A master's program offered in Athens in Greece by the branch campus of the University of Indianapolis that is fully owned and controlled by its U.S. parent. The program is accredited by the Higher Learning Commission of the North Central Association of Colleges and Schools. The program is taught by experienced educators with professional backgrounds.

Faculty Research
NP

100% faculty in professional counseling practice.

Degree Programs

Degree	Program	Contact
BSc	Psychology	
MA	Clincal Psychology/Mental Health Counseling	

Distance learning: N; 0% courses on-line

Faculty

Name		Highest Degree	Rank	Email
Rein	Ron	PhD	Assistant Professor	reinr@uindy.gr
Rush	Anastasia	PhD	Professor	rusha@uindy.gr
Schina	Margarita	PhD	Assistant Professor	schinam@uindy.gr
Simoglou	Vassiliki	DEA, MA	Senior Lecturer	simoglouv@uindy.gr

Enrollment and Admission Requirements

Degree	Program	Enrollment and Admission
BSc	Psychology	
MA	Clincal Psychology/Mental Health Counseling	First Degree - (in Psychology, or if in another discipline, foundation course requirement on entry). GRE requirement if GPA <3.0. English proficiency.

Graduation Requirements

Degree	Program	Duration	Practicum	Internship	Thesis/ Dissertation	Comp	Oral	Portfolio
BSc	Psychology Internship optional	4 years		Y	N	Y	N	N
MA	Clincal Psychology/Mental Health Counseling	2-5 years		Y	Y	Y	N	N

The curriculum is designed to meet the requirements for graduate study specified in Indiana State laws regulating the licensing of Mental Health Counselors.

GUATEMALA: Universidad del Valle de Guatemala

18 Avenida 11-95 Zona 15 Vista Hermosa III
Guatemala 01015
Guatemala
www.uvg.edu.gt

Dean	Dra. Cristina de Luj
	18 Avenida 11-95 Zona 15
	Vista Hermosa III
	Guatemala 01015
	Guatemala
Administrator	Donald A Prentice, Ing.
	18 Avenida 11-95 Zona 15
	Vista Hermosa III
	Guatemala 01015
	Guatemala
	telephone: 011 502 23690791; fax: 011 502 23649952
	daprentice@uvg.edu.gt

Regionally Accredited NP
Financial Aid NP

Program Uniqueness

The program has been co-constructed through international collaboration and has a community multicultural emphasis from an integrative perspective. It is the first program in Guatemala.

Faculty Research

Counseling training, supervision, and counseling process; gender and cultural issues; prevention and wellness; mental health.

40% faculty in professional counseling practice.

Degree Programs

Degree	*Program*	*Contact*
Magister Atrium M.A.	Maestría en Consejería Psicológica y Salud Mental	
Magister Atrium M.A.	Maestría en Consejería Psicológica y Salud Mental	

Distance learning: Y; 10% courses on-line

Faculty
NP

Enrollment and Admission Requirements

Degree	Program	Enrollment and Admission Requirement
Magister Atrium M.A.	Maestría en Consejería Psicológica y Salud Mental	Licenciatura Degree or the equivalent in credit hours (58 credit hours of a finished undergraduate degree)
Magister Atrium M.A.	Maestría en Consejería Psicológica y Salud Mental	Licenciatura Degree or the equivalent in credit hours (58 credit hours of a finished undergraduate degree)

Graduation Requirements

Degree	Program	Duration	Practicum	Internship	Thesis/ Dissertation	Comp	Oral	Portfolio
Magister Atrium M.A.	Maestría en Consejería Psicológica y Salud Mental	36 months		Y	Y	N	Y	Y
Magister Atrium M.A.	Maestría en Consejería Psicológica y Salud Mental	36 months		Y	Y	N	Y	Y

The students prior to graduation need to either present at a congress/conference or academic meeting or publish a manuscript in an academic/professional publication.

ITALY: Libera Universita` del Counseling - Free University of Counseling

Castello della Rancia - Tolentino
Tolentino (MC) 62029
Italy
www.unicouns.it

Dean   Professor - Director Vincenzo Masini
Via Romana number 1189
Lucca Tuscany, 55100
Italy

Administrator   Vincenzo Masini, Professor
Via Romana number 1189
Lucca Tuscany, 55100
Italy
telephone: +39 3355475302; fax: NP
prepos@prepos.it

Regionally Accredited NP
Financial Aid   NP

Program Uniqueness

The innovative dimension of the Free University of Counseling is the sharing of the best counselor education available in Italy by connecting different models and schools of counseling, and creating the relational way of the counseling profession.

Faculty Research
NP

% faculty in professional counseling practice: NP

Degree Programs
NP

Distance learning: N; 0% courses on-line: NP

Faculty
NP

Enrollment and Admission Requirements

NP

Graduation Requirements
NP

KENYA: Kenya Association of Professional Counsellors

55472
Nairobi 00200
Kenya
www.kapc.or.ke

Dean	Cecilia Rachier (M.S.), Executive Director
	55472
	Nairobi 00200
	Kenya
Administrator	Elias Gikundi, Deputy Executive Director
	55472
	Nairobi 00200
	Kenya
	telephone: 3741051; fax: 3741051
	egikundi@kapc.or.ke

Regionally Accredited NP
Financial Aid   NP

Program Uniqueness

Our program is very practical, experiential and community-oriented.

Faculty Research

Education, HIV/AIDS, Gender, Sexuality, Marriage and Family.

80% faculty in professional counseling practice.

Degree Programs

Degree	*Program*	*Contact*
X	BA in Counselling Studies	Cecilia Rachier
Master	2 years	

Distance learning: Y; 10% courses on-line

Faculty
NP

Enrollment and Admission Requirements

Degree	*Program*	*Enrollment and Admission Requirement*
X	B.A. in Counselling Studies	12 years of Education, Aggregate C+ Counselling Certificate Essential
Master	2 years	At least a first degree in helping area.

Graduation Requirements

Degree	Program	Duration	Practicum	Internship	Thesis/ Dissertation	Comp	Oral	Portfolio
X	B.A. in Counselling Studies	Two week blocks 3 years		N	Y		Y	Y
Master		2 years		N	Y	Y	Y	Y
	Available in the East and South Africa Region							

NIGERIA: Alvan Ikoku Federal College of Education [UNN Counselling Programme]

PMB 1033
Owerri 234
Nigeria

Dean   NP

Administrator   NP

Regionally Accredited NP
Financial Aid   NP

Program Uniqueness
NP

Faculty Research
NP

% faculty in professional counseling practice: NP

Degree Programs
NP

Distance learning: NP; NP % courses on-line

Faculty
NP

Enrollment and Admission Requirements

NP

Graduation Requirements
NP

NIGERIA: Ibrahim Badamasi Babangida University

P.M.B. 11
Lapai 234
Nigeria
nil

Dean   Mrs. V.I. Ezenwa, Professor
Faculty of Education and Arts
Ibrahim Badamasi Babangida University
Lapai 234
Nigeria

Administrator   Dr. George Bamidele Ewenyi
Faculty of Education and Arts
Ibrahim Badamasi Babangida University
Lapai, 234
Nigeria
telephone: 2348032953889; fax: NIL
georgeeweniyi@yahoo.co.uk

Regionally Accredited NP
Financial Aid   NP

Program Uniqueness

The programme is unique because it concentrates on producing counselling psychologists for schools and other aspects of the national economy.

Faculty Research
NP

% faculty in professional counseling practice: NP

Degree Programs

Degree	Program	Contact
B.Ed	B.Ed. (Counselling Psychology)	

Distance learning: N; 0% courses on-line

Faculty
NP

Enrollment and Admission Requirements

Degree	Program	Enrollment and Admission Requirement
B.Ed	B.Ed (Counselling Psychology)	General requirements: Candidates must satisfy the IBB University's minimum entry qualifications which stipulate 5 credits including English language and mathematics in GCE/SSCE O level, NECO/WAEC (in not more than two sittings). UME requirements:(4 Year B.Ed Counselling Psychology): Candidates apart from the University requirements must have at least credit passes in literature-in-English and any other 2 arts, social science or science subjects. Direct entry (3 Year B.Ed Counselling Psychology Programme): Must satisfy the general O level requirements of the university. In addition, candidates must have at least credit passes in English/literature-in-English and any other 2 arts subjects at the Advanced Level GCE, or at Principal level in the HSC examination, N.C.E. or IJMB examination.

Graduation Requirements

Degree	Program	Duration	Practicum	Internship	Thesis/ Dissertation	Comp	Oral	Portfolio
B.Ed	B.Ed (Counselling Psychology)	4 years		Y	Y	Y	N	

NIGERIA: LAGOS STATE UNIVERSITY

	PMB 0001, LASU Post Office Badagry Expressway Lagos +234 Nigeria
Dean	N.C. Nwaboku, Professor Faculty of Education PMB 0001, LASU Post Office Badagry Expressway Lagos +234 Nigeria
Administrator	E.A. Akinade, Professor of Counselling Psychology Faculty of Education Lagos State University PMB 0001, LASU Post Office Badagry Expressway Lagos +234 Nigeria telephone: +2348033370697 and +233543010007; fax: NP emanuelalasu@yahoo.com

Regionally Accredited NP
Financial Aid NP

Program Uniqueness

We train higher degree students to be consultants in grief and retirement counselling.

Faculty Research

Retirement and grief counselling; stress management; counselling people with special needs; vocational development; and strategies for reducing drug abuse.

35% faculty in professional counseling practice.

Degree Programs
NP

Distance learning: N; 0% courses on-line

Faculty
NP

Enrollment and Admission Requirements
NP

Graduation Requirements
NP

NIGERIA: University of Lagos

Department of Educational Foundations
Lagos 0234
Nigeria
www.unilag.edu.ng

Dean   Professor Bidmos
Faculty of Education
University of Lagos
Akoka - Lagos 0234
Nigeria

Administrator   Olusakin Ayoka Mopelola, Professor
Faculty of Education
University of Lagos
Akoka - Lagos 0234
Nigeria
telephone: 2348033043979; fax: NP
mopeolusakin@yahoo.com

Regionally Accredited NP
Financial Aid   NP

Program Uniqueness
NP

Faculty Research

Adolescents and youths counseling, university students counseling, marital counseling, and pastoral counselling.

100% faculty in professional counseling practice.

Degree Programs

Degree	Program	Contact
B.A (Ed.) Guidance & Counselling	Undergraduate Degree in Guidance and Counselling	Admissions Office, University of Lagos
M.Ed Guidance & Counselling	Masters in Guidance & Counselling	School of Postgraduate Studies, University of Lagos
Ph.D in Guidance & Counselling	Doctor of Philosophy in Guidance & Counselling	School of Postgraduate Studies, University of Lagos

Distance learning: N; 5% courses on-line

Faculty

Name		Highest Degree	Rank	Email
Olusakin	Ayoka Mopelola	Ph.D. in Counselling Psychology	Professor	mopeolusakin@yahoo.com

Enrollment and Admission Requirements

Degree	Program	Enrollment and Admission Requirement
B.A (Ed.) Guidance & Counselling	Undergraduate Degree in Guidance and Counselling	Minimum of five credits (at one sitting) in arts subjects inclusive of English language and mathematics.
M.Ed. Guidance & Counselling	Master's in Guidance & Counselling	A good first degree in Education or PGDE from a recognised University.
Ph.D. in Guidance & Counselling	Doctor of Philosophy in Guidance & Counselling	Masters in Guidance & Counselling with a minimum Cumulative Grade Point of 4.0 for Ph.D.

Graduation Requirements

Degree	Program	Duration	Practicum	Internship	Thesis/ Dissertation	Comp	Oral	Portfolio
B.A (Ed) Guidance & Counselling	Undergraduate Degree in Guidance and Counselling	40 months -3 years (Direct Entry) or 4 sessions		Y	Y	Y		
	Sandwich Programmes available for minimum of 5 (Direct Entry) or 6 sessions.							
M.Ed (Guidance & Counselling)	Master's in Guidance & Counselling	12 months		Y	Y	Y		
	Sandwich programme is available for 2 sessions.							
Ph.D. in Guidance & Counselling	Doctor of Philosophy in Guidance & Counselling	30 Months Minimum of 3 sessions		Y	Y	Y	Y	

ROMANIA: University of Bucharest

36-46 M.Kogalniceanu Bd sector 5
Bucharest, Romania 70709
Romania

Dean

Dr. Neculai Mitrofan, Professor
Faculty of Psychology and Sciences of Education
1-3 Iuliu Maniu
Corp A, et. 5
Bucharest 70709
Romania

Administrator

Gheorghe Tomsa, Professor
1-3 Iuliu Maniu
Bucharest 70709
Romania
telephone: 0040744494196; fax: 0040213181550
gheorghetomsa@yahoo.com

Regionally Accredited NP
Financial Aid NP

Program Uniqueness

This program was the first Master`s in Counseling (School Counseling) organized in Romania in 1996.

Faculty Research
NP

0% faculty in professional counseling practice.

Degree Programs

Degree	Program	Contact
Master	Integrative Education	Gheorghe Tomsa
MEd	School Counseling	Gheorghe Tomsa

Distance learning: Y; NP% courses on-line

Faculty

Name		Highest Degree	Rank	Email
Bonciu	Catalina	PhD	Full Professor	catalina_ioana.bonciu@unibuc.ro
Iucu	Romita	PhD	Full Professor, Vice Rector	romiuc@yahoo.com
Mitrofan	Nicolae	PhD	Professor and Associate Dean	nmitrofan@hotmail.com
Mitrofan	Iolanda	PhD	Full Professor	nmitrofan@hotmail.com
Neacsu	Ioan	PHD	Full Professor	
Potolea	Dan	PhD	Academic Dean & Professor	dpotolea@yahoo.com
Szilagyi	Andreea	PhD	Visiting Associate Professor	szilagyi@nbcc.ro
Tomsa	Gheorghe	CAGS	Full Professor & Director of the Master's Program	gheorghetomsa@yahoo.com
Verza	Emil	PHD	Full Professor	
Vrasmas	Ecaterina	PhD	Full Professor	ecaterinavr@yahoo.com

Enrollment and Admission Requirements

Degree	Program	Enrollment and Admission Requirement
Master	Integrative Education	
MEd	School Counseling	

Graduation Requirements

Degree	Program	Duration	Practicum	Internship	Thesis/ Dissertation	Comp	Oral	Portfolio
Master	Integrative Education	2 years			Y			Y
MEd	School Counseling				Y			

UNITED KINGDOM: Academy of Play & Child Psychotherapy

NP
http://www.apac.org.uk/

Dean	Monika Jephcott, Programme Director The Coach House Belmont Road Uckfield East Sussex TN22 1BP United Kingdom
Administrator	Linda Bradley, Course Administrator The Coach House Belmont Road Uckfield East Sussex TN22 1BP United Kingdom telephone: +44 (0)1825 761143; fax: NP mokijep@aol.com

Regionally Accredited NP
Financial Aid NP

Program Uniqueness

The only Master's programme for play therapy validated by clinical outcome research.

Faculty Research
NP

% faculty in professional counseling practice: NP

Degree Programs

Degree	*Program*	*Contact*
Master	M.A. in Practice Based Play Therapy	Monika Jephcott

Distance learning: N; 0% courses on-line

Faculty: NP

Enrollment and Admission Requirements

Degree	*Program*	*Enrollment and Admission Requirements*
Master	M.A. in Practice Based Play Therapy	Bachelor's in psychology, child care, teaching or a related subject, or a professional Diploma. At least 2 years experience of working with children.

Graduation Requirements

Degree	Program	Duration	Practicum	Internship	Thesis/ Dissertation	Comp	Oral	Portfolio
Master	M.A. in Practice Based Play Therapy	3 to 5 years		Y	Y	N	N	Y

The programme is delivered in three stages: Post Graduate Certificate in Therapeutic Play, Post Graduate Diploma in Play Therapy, and M.A. in Practice Based Play Therapy (by dissertation). Students may exit at any stage.

VENEZUELA: The University of Zulia

Av. 16 Goajira
Maracaibo Zulia 4015
Venezuela (Bolivarian Republic of)
http://www.postgradofhe.com/

Dean   Dean Dra. Doris Sala
Av. Goajira. Facultad de Humanidades y Educacion
Maracaibo Zulia 4015
Venezuela (Bolivarian Republic of)

Administrator   Dr. Rexne Castro, Director
Av. Goajira. Facultad de Humanidades y Educacion
Graduate Studies Building
Maracaibo Zulia 4015
Venezuela (Bolivarian Republic of)
telephone: (58) 2617590824

Regionally Accredited NP
Financial Aid   NP

Program Uniqueness

One of the oldest and most prestigious universities in the country.

Faculty Research

College Counseling.

% faculty in professional counseling practice: NP

Degree Programs

Degree	Program	Contact
Bachelors degree in Education, Major: Counseling	Undergraduate	Dr. Luz Maldonado
Master of Science in Counseling Major: Educational Counseling or Workplace Counseling	Graduate Degree Program	Dr. George Davy Vera

Distance learning: N; 0% courses on-line

Faculty

Name		Highest Degree	Rank	Email
Campo	Maria Susana	Doctorate in Human Science	Professor	auramarlara@hotmail.com
Dolores	Maria	Master Science in Counseling	Professor	lunezca@yahoo.com
Herrera	Mireya	Master Science in Counseling	Professor	mireya1205@gmail.com
Jimenez	Dorelys	PhD Counselor Education	Professor	dorelys61@yahoo.com
Maldonado	Luz	Doctorate in Counseling	Professor	luzmercedesmaldonado@hotmail.com
Vargas	Aura	Master Science in Counseling	Professor	auramarlara@hotmail.com
Vera	George	PhD Counselor Education	Professor	gdavyvera@gmail.com
Villa	Gabriel	Doctorate in Education	Professor	gabrielvillae@gmail.com
Zamora	Maigualida	Doctorate in Human Science	Professor	maigualidaz@gmail.com

Enrollment and Admission Requirements

Degree	Program	Enrollment and Admission Requirement
Bachelors degree in Education, Major: Counseling	Undergraduate	1. High school Diploma. 2. Admission evaluation.
Master of Science in Counseling, Major: Educational Counseling or Workplace Counseling	Graduate Degree Program	1. A proper bachelor's degree in Education, Psychology, Social Work, Counseling, Medicine or Sociology. 2. Approved admission evaluation test.

Graduation Requirements

Degree	Program	Duration	Practicum	Internship	Thesis/ Dissertation	Comp	Oral	Portfolio
Bachelors degree in Education, Major: Counseling	Undergraduate	5 years		Y	N	N		Y
	600 hours of continuing counseling pre-services under qualified supervision.							
Master of Science in Counseling, Major: Educational Counseling or Workplace Counseling	Graduate Degree Program	2 years		N	Y			

Faculty Index